A Small Guide To
Losing Big

From the Nutritionist for NBC's *The Biggest Loser*

CHERYL FORBERG, R.D.

Notice

This book is intended as a reference volume only, not as a medical manual. The information given here is designed to help you make informed decisions about your health. It is not intended as a substitute for any treatment that may have been prescribed by your doctor. If you suspect that you have a medical problem, we urge you to seek competent medical help. The information in this book is meant to supplement, not replace, proper exercise training. All forms of exercise pose some inherent risks. The editors and publisher advise readers to take full responsibility for their safety and know their limits. Before practicing the exercises in this book, be sure that your equipment is well-maintained, and do not take risks beyond your level of experience, aptitude, training and fitness. The exercise and dietary programs in this book are not intended as a substitute for any exercise routine or dietary regimen that may have been prescribed by your doctor. As with all exercise and dietary programs, you should get your doctor's approval before beginning.

Mention of specific companies, organizations or authorities in this book does not imply endorsement by the author or publisher, nor does mention of specific companies, organizations or authorities imply that they endorse this book, its author or the publisher.

Internet addresses and telephone numbers given in this book were accurate at the time it went to press.

Flavor First LLC books may be purchased for business or promotional use or for special sales. For information, please write to: Special Markets Department, Flavor First LLC, P.O. Box 6554, Napa, CA 94581 or media@flavorfirst.com

Printed in China by Global PSD, www.GlobalPSD.com

Book design Kevin Evans
Back flap photo by Neely Wang Photography
Library of Congress Cataloging-in-Publication Data
Forberg, Cheryl

ISBN- 978-0-9908122-0-3

10 9 8 7 6 5 4 3 2 1 paperback

A Small Guide To
Losing Big

From the Nutritionist for NBC's *The Biggest Loser*

CHERYL FORBERG, R.D.

This book is dedicated to my incredible clients — those I've worked with privately and those who have shared their stories as contestants on NBC's The Biggest Loser. I wish I could list each of you by name. You were with me in spirit as I wrote every page. I cannot thank you enough for allowing me to participate in your transformation and life's journey. You have each touched me personally and, for that, you are truly the inspiration for this book.

Table of Contents

Introduction

After 15 seasons as the nutritionist for NBC's *The Biggest Loser*, I've learned a great deal about the typical eating habits of many Americans, particularly the habits that cause weight gain. When I sit down with my clients or with the contestants at the Ranch for a one-on-one nutrition consultation, we review their food journals and I help them understand how their food choices - both good and bad - impact their waistlines and their overall health.

Oftentimes, they're shocked to discover how many calories they've been taking in, as well as the unlikely sources of those extra calories. Some clients and contestants are stunned to learn that they've been consuming an entire day's worth of calories in their beverages alone, while others discover that the seemingly "healthful choices" they've been making aren't nearly as nutritious or as low in calories as they'd assumed.

Many of my clients and contestants are reluctant to part with their highly processed favorites because they don't think their cravings can be satisfied with "healthful food." But it's a misconception that simple, nutritious foods can't be absolutely loaded with flavor. And that's a very big part of this book. In addition to sharing my winning weight-loss advice, I'm also sharing two weeks of menus and 25 recipes to get you started. For more recipes, please visit my website, cherylforberg.com.

From your starting calorie budget, shopping list, meal plans and recipes, to exercises for your physical (and emotional) health - everything you need is in your hands. And because I'm a chef *and* a dietitian, you'll also learn how to enhance and coax the natural, delicious flavors from fresh foods in a minimal amount of time and effort.
Let's get started!

Chapter One:
The *Losing Big* Overview

Change Your Habits, Change Your Life

For many of us, weight gain - and, ultimately, effective weight management - is about more than what we eat. Emotions, hormones, busy schedules and finances affect the everyday choices we make. And as the pounds pile up, it can be frustrating and confusing to get off that slippery slope and back on track again.

One thing I've heard over and over from my clients and *Biggest Loser* contestants is this: Collectively, they had tried just about every crazy diet out there but have found that my plan works. Why? Instead of blindly following an "eat this, don't eat that" type of plan, they understand why they are being asked to make certain choices. If you are like many of my clients, a really important part of the process for you will be in taking the time to learn the key underlying principles to effective nutrition and weight management. When a nutritional plan makes sense, it's easier to knowingly - rather than blindly - follow it.

This plan works! Just ask 15 seasons of big losers and hundreds of my clients! But the plan will work only if you make the commitment to break your eating patterns, change the way you think about food, and replace your bad habits with a few simple good ones. This will help manage your weight - and health - for the rest of your life! It's important to note that the style of eating I recommend is not only for the obese or those struggling with weight management. The menus and recipes are great for everyone wanting to eat more healthfully. I encourage you to share them with friends and family, too.

Here's the rub, though. Most people, no matter how badly they want to lose weight, are just too busy to read an entire book cover to cover - they pick and choose the parts of a book that are most meaningful to them and leave the rest. That sometimes can mean inadvertently omitting really important information.

This book is a simple solution for people who are busy... like you!

The most effective and powerful advice I've given over the years has been culled and simplified in this handy, portable, easy-to-read (and easy to remember!), step-by-step guide. But if you're the type (like many of my friends and family members) who wants to begin *without* having to start on page one, I've included a jumpstart plan on page 9 that will point you to the most critical steps in the process.

My hope is that you will refer to it over and over again, and share these basics with your friends and family, too. I promise you'll experience increased energy, better sleep and weight loss. The more you do, the more results you'll see and feel.

As with all exercise and dietary programs, you should get your doctor's approval before beginning. The tests your health provider orders will depend on your history. Generally, your work-up will include a blood pressure check, a blood test and, sometimes, urinalysis. Ask your doctor which biomarker exams may be beneficial to you (see *Appendix 3* for recommended biomarker tests). Be sure to record all values in a journal to serve as your baseline. You can track your progress over weeks, months and years.

The *Losing Big* Jumpstart Plan

Ready to get started without having to start on page one?
Use this handy jumpstart plan that will point you
to the most critical steps in the process.

1. Calculate Your Daily Calories Needs - Page 13

2. Set Up Your Journal - Page 15

3. Measure/Test Your Biomarkers - Appendix 3, Page 130

4. Answer This - Are You an Emotional Eater? - Page 19

5. Divvy Up Your Daily Calorie Budget - Page 31

6. Choose Right Foods - Page 36, Food List - Page 90

7. Shop - Page 62

8. Customize Your Exercise Regimen - Page 51

9. Cook - Page 74

10. SOS! When You're Feeling Stuck - Page 80

11. Manage Your Plan Away From Home

    • At the Office - Page 83
    • Eating Out - Page 85
    • On the Road - Page 86
    • Navigating Holidays and Special Events - Page 89

12. Two Weeks of *Losing Big* Menus
    and 25 Scrumptious Recipes - Page 97

Chapter Two:
How Many Calories Do I Need in a Day?

A Calorie by Any Other Name...

Calorie. For many of you the mere word can conjure up a host of feelings and emotions - perhaps many of them negative. If you're reading this book, it's likely you've spent a good portion of your life thinking about calories on a daily basis. A 2011 U.S. Gallup poll found that 23% of men and 37% of women have tried to lose weight between 3 and 10 times throughout their lives.[1] In Britain, a recent poll of 2,000 adults found that more than 75% had tried a diet in the past year and, likewise, more than 75% try a different diet every two months.[2] If you're lucky enough that you haven't had to think about calories until now - you must have been doing something right!

Understanding what calories are and how they contribute to your body's energy system is necessary to knowing how to adequately fuel your body, balance calories in and calories out, and manage your overall health and weight.

Let's Start with the Basics

A *calorie* (also called a *kilocalorie*) is a unit of energy, technically the amount of energy needed to raise the temperature of 1 gram of water by 1 degree Celsius. Calories provide the fuel your body uses to produce energy, powering your body much in the same way that gasoline powers a car.

Most foods are a blend of protein, fat and carbs, and each component contributes a set number of calories per gram. *Fats* contain 9 calories per gram, *proteins* 4 calories per gram, and *carbohydrates* 4 calories per gram. (Alcohol contains calories, too. Pure alcohol carries 7 calories per gram!) The number of calories in everything you eat or drink is a measure of the stored energy in that food - the amount of energy available to your body from the foods that you eat. And *metabolism* - a set of chemical reactions in our bodies - is the breaking down of food to create energy (catabolism) and the usage of that energy to construct our cells (anabolism). Your metabolic rate is a measure of the speed of your metabolism - the rate at which your body converts what you eat and drink into energy.

Some foods are nutrient-dense, which means you're getting the most nutrient bang for calorie buck. For instance, 10 calories worth of fresh tomato has much more nutritional value than 10 soft drink calories. Whether rich or poor in nutrients, calories that you consume but don't burn off are stored in your body as reserve energy. Can you guess how these extra calories are stored? Yep, as fat. In order to burn off that reserve energy store called fat, you need to eat or drink fewer calories than you burn through physical activity.

Simple, right?

Not so fast! Everyone's body burns (metabolizes) calories at a different rate. Even when resting, your body needs energy for breathing, circulating blood, heartbeat, adjusting hormone levels, and growing and repairing cells. Your resting metabolic rate (RMR) is the number of calories *your* body needs to fuel these basic energy needs in a 24-hour period. Several factors contribute to individual metabolic rate:

- Body size and amount of muscle mass. People who are larger or who have more muscle burn more calories, even when they're resting.

- Gender. Men typically have less body fat and more muscle than women of the same age and weight, and thus burn more calories.

- Age. As we age, the amount of muscle we have naturally tends to decrease, leaving fat to account for more of our weight, slowing the calorie-burning process even further.[3]

Approximately 60% to 75% of the calories you take in each day go directly to support RMR functions. Our bodies are well-tuned to keep things at status quo. In addition, a small percentage of the calories you consume are sucked up by food digestion (it's true, digesting food burns calories!) and the rest are allocated to help you get through your daily routine. The trick is in calculating what your body requires, then balancing calorie intake and output. Easier said than done! But that's why you're reading this book.

Optimal Calorie Burn: The REAL X Factor

The variable factor in determining how many calories you burn in a day - and the one you have the most control over - is your level of physical activity, both in intensity and duration. Muscles burn a lot of calories even when you're at rest, but, sadly, muscles shrink with age. And as they shrink, your body will burn fewer and fewer calories.

Dehydration: Did you know?

In hot weather your body is prone to dehydration, and this can have a devastating effect on your metabolism. In the course of an average day your sweating, breathing, and waste elimination can leach more than 10 cups of water out of your body, and that's without exercise! Because blood is mostly water, dehydration can cause the volume of your blood to diminish, lowering amounts of oxygen and nutrients that need to reach your tissues, slowing your metabolism, and causing you to burn fewer calories. Dehydration can also sap your body's energy levels, affecting your desire or ability to exercise, a dehydration double whammy. If you're exercising in hot weather, be sure to drink plenty of water to stay hydrated!

Exercise - both resistance training and cardio work - is an important component of overall health and, specifically, weight loss. We will discuss the details of exercise and the importance of building and maintaining muscle mass, particularly to counteract the natural loss of muscle during aging, in *Chapter Seven, Burn and Build - Exercise for Weight Loss*.

Calculating Your Calorie Needs

There are a couple of quick ways to estimate your calorie needs for long-term weight-loss success, but *be sure to maintain a minimum of 1,200 calories per day.*

The following is for calculating the estimated calories needed for weight maintenance. For weight loss, subtract 500 calories from the end number.

- *For less-active individuals*:
  Weight (in pounds) x 14 = estimated calories/day.

- *For moderately active individuals* (3 to 4 aerobic sessions/week):
  Weight (in pounds) x 17 = estimated calories/day.

- *For active individuals* (5 to 7 aerobic sessions/week):
  Weight (in pounds) x 20 = estimated calories/day.

- *If you really want to skip the calculations*: Lopping 500 calories off your daily intake is a good place to start if you want to lose about a pound per week.

For information on how to estimate calories in food and read nutritional labels, go to *Chapter Eight, Stocking Your Kitchen*, Page 64, *Deciphering Food Labels*.

Keep in mind, though, that we all burn calories at different rates due to differences in age, gender and body composition. If you're following this plan with a buddy, the two of you may lose weight at different rates. And your own weight loss will likely vary from week to week. Don't let that derail you! This is completely normal. Consistent effort over time is what ensures a lifetime of good health.

For those of you looking to fine-tune your caloric intake and expenditures for losing (or, in some circumstances, gaining) weight, the Harris Benedict

Equation can be used for calculating your basal metabolic rate (BMR) and caloric needs. Refer to Appendix 3, *Basal Metabolic Rate Biomarker* (Page 141) for BMR calculations. Note your Daily Calorie Needs/Goal in your Food Journal, and update it as you lose weight and adjust your calorie needs.

Adjusting Calorie Needs

I know this is going to surprise some of you, but as you lose weight, your daily calorie intake may need to... drop! That can be a shocker, but don't panic. Although we're not talking about significant additional calorie cutting, you will need to tweak your calorie intake as you drop weight.

Why? It takes a lot of energy to move body weight around. Bigger bodies – whether fat or fit - burn more calories than smaller bodies. As you lose weight, your relatively smaller body may need fewer calories. For every pound of fat you lose, you will burn around 10 fewer calories each day - roughly the number of calories (energy) needed to maintain that pound of fat and support its metabolic needs. So when you drop 10 pounds, you will burn approximately 100 fewer calories each day than you did when you weighed more. That means you will need to make adjustments if you want to continue to lose weight.

The good news is that once you reach your weight-loss goal, you may slowly begin to add quality calories back into your daily routine to find the right calorie in/calorie out formula for your weight-maintenance balance point. Everyone is different, so pay attention to your energy and hunger levels.

Chapter Three
Food Journaling - Critical to Weight-Loss Success

Put Your Mind to It -
Knuckle Down, Buckle Down, Do it, Do it, DO IT![4]

When trying to lose weight, it's critical that you pay attention to - and are mindful of - everything you eat and drink. It sounds simple enough, right? Mindful eating is something we should all do, but all too often we, well, forget.

And according to researchers at the University of Birmingham in England who conducted a study on mindful eating, the effects of an unmemorable meal reach well beyond a wasted lunch.

Researchers fed three groups of women identical lunches. One group ate with nothing but their lunches to keep them occupied. A second group read a newspaper article on changes in chocolate bar sizes and soft drinks while eating. The third group ate while listening to audio instructions on how to focus on the look, smell, flavors and textures of their food.

An hour later, researchers served the women plates of sweets.

The group encouraged via audio instructions to focus on their food *ate 50% to 60% fewer sweets* than the two groups who ate mindlessly! Researchers concluded that the group who focused on their food ate less when offered sweets because *they retained the most vivid memory of their meals.*[5]

What can we learn from this? Stopping to appreciate each bite of food - how the flavors work together, what textures are at play, and even how your food looks - is important not just to your overall enjoyment of your meals but also to your waistline. When you eat mindfully - *noticing, appreciating, and savoring* your food - you feel full longer. And feeling full can make it easier to stick to your calorie budget.

Help for the Mindless - Keep a Food Journal

All of us eat mindlessly from time to time and can suffer from food amnesia - "forgetting" that we've had nibbles, snacks, drinks or even an entire meal. And a nibble or two here and there can add up to hundreds of calories in a day's time. Plus, for some, it's not just hunger that drives us to the fridge; many of us may have emotional triggers that cause us to eat (see *Chapter Four, Emotional Eating* for more information).

A food journal can help you identify when and why you eat certain things, and help you learn from your eating patterns. Perhaps more importantly, knowing that you have to record every morsel and every sip you put in your mouth just might make you think twice before mindlessly munching on foods that can undermine your weight-loss efforts!

One of the first tasks I give my clients - including Biggest Loser contestants - is to *write down everything they put into their mouths*. Oftentimes they're shocked to discover how many calories they've been taking in. They can look up their calories in a calorie counter book, or use one of the many available online sources.

I can't deny it can be a pain in the beginning, but most of us are creatures of habit, eating the same meals and snacks more than one time in a week. After a week or two, the process will actually be something you can look forward to as you begin to observe how much you can control your weight destiny by being accountable.

After experiencing how incredibly effective journaling is for weight loss/maintenance, most vow to maintain this practice for life. But life happens and some fall off the journaling wagon. I still get calls from clients and *Biggest Loser* contestants I haven't seen in years who tell me if the pounds start to come back, the first thing they do is pull out their food journals and a pen.

Mind Your Food (and Your Butt Will Follow)!

Not convinced? Then consider this. A 2008 study, one of the largest and longest-running weight loss maintenance trials ever conducted, found that dieters who kept food journals at least six days a week lost twice as much weight as those who journaled one day a week or not at all.

And in 2012, a study of 123 previously inactive, overweight, postmenopausal women – half of whom exercised and followed a calorie-restricted diet while the other half only dieted – found that while both groups lost an average of 10% of their starting weight at the end of one year, the women who consistently used food journals lost approximately 6 pounds more than those who didn't! Also, those who skipped meals lost significantly less weight, on average, than those who ate regularly scheduled snacks and meals.[6] (*See Chapter Five, When Can I Eat?* for more details on when to eat.)

It's simple. Once you've established your daily calorie budget (see *Chapter Two, How Many Calories Do I Need?*) make time to record your food, beverages and exercise daily. Keeping a food journal will help you fine-tune your eating strategy, pace meals and snacks, and identify satisfying foods. For a sample food journal page, see Appendix 4, page 147.

Tips for successful journaling:

- *Make it easy*. Buy a notebook that's small enough to go anywhere and keep it, and a pen, with you. If you're a techie, find a mobile app that helps you track food on the go. (*See Web Resources* page 155)

- *Be fanatical.* Starting first thing in the morning, write down everything you eat and drink (including water), noting the time.

- *Quantify.* Weigh and measure food when you can, or estimate quantities and include with your entry. (See *Chapter Nine, Cooking Tools and Techniques.*)

- *Calories count.* Be sure to include calorie counts and keep a running count throughout the day. You don't want to get to dinnertime with only 50 calories left to spend!

- *Assess your hunger.* Quantify and record your level of hunger before AND after eating (see page 30 for the Hunger Scale). Some people need the feeling of being full. Note in your journal if you're still hungry after a meal, then divvy up your calories differently the next day. Write it in your journal, and note if that helped you feel satisfied.

- *Let yourself feel.* Jot down emotions - including how food you ate made you feel. If you binged (it happens!), try to identify what caused it (did you receive bad news and head straight for the fridge?). If you had an epiphany and didn't need food, analyze why. This is really important.

- *Snap a photo.* Too busy to write things down? Snap a pic with your phone, then record the foods (and feelings) in your journal at night.

- *Keep track of exercise.* Include scheduled workouts and any incidental exercise (like walking the dog or playing catch with your child).

- *Be mindful of being mindful!* Note everything from the cream in your morning coffee (please use milk!) to your bowl of frozen yogurt at midnight.

- *Analyze your journal each day.* Notice patterns in your behavior, determine problem areas and make adjustments.

Chapter Four
Emotional Eating

When Food Replaces Feelings

Let's face it, for most of us, food is more than merely fuel for our bodies - much more. From Grandma's apple pie to mac and cheese we enjoyed as a child to chocolate mousse shared with a love, food can evoke memories and emotions, particularly feelings of comfort or love.

But there's a big difference between nurturing yourself from time to time with comfort food, and using food to insulate you from your feelings and emotions. When eating becomes a method of self-medicating - or numbing yourself to feelings - emotional eating crosses over into the realm of concern. Over the years I've learned that understanding and addressing the emotional aspects of overeating and weight management are just as important as nutrition and exercise.

*Emotional eating is reaching for food
to quell feelings, rather than hunger.*

While my plan is simple, following it can be a challenge if you've fallen out of touch with your body's hunger cues and developed bad habits or an unhealthy routine. Emotional eating doesn't help either. (For more on hunger cues, see the Hunger Scale in *Chapter Five, When Can I Eat?*)

Identifying Emotional vs. Physical Hunger

Stress, anxiety, loneliness and fatigue are common triggers for emotional eaters, particularly women. If one of your happiest moments growing up with your six siblings was sitting at the kitchen table eating Mom's spaghetti with tomato sauce, you may crave pasta when you're feeling lonely or blue.

But differentiating physical hunger and emotional hunger can be difficult, especially if you've spent your life stuffing your emotions by reaching for food.

Tips on recognizing emotional eating:

- *Emotional hunger comes on suddenly.* Physical hunger typically comes on gradually... and you may have physical signs like your stomach growling, for instance.

- *Emotional hunger craves specific - in most cases, unhealthful - foods.* When you're physically hungry, almost anything will do, including healthful foods.

- *Emotional hunger results in mindless eating.* Just consumed a pint of ice cream before bed without realizing or enjoying it? Just polished off a sleeve of cookies in front of the television after work? Inhaled a drive-thru burger while crawling home in rush-hour traffic? These instances are most likely emotional eating.

- *Emotional hunger is never satiated.* You want more and more, eating until you're stuffed (often referred to as Carb Coma).

- *Emotional hunger has repercussions.* Guilt, shame, regret - to name a few. Physical hunger never leaves you feeling badly about yourself.[7]

While most of us - at one time or another during our lives - have used food for something *other* than feeding hunger, some grapple with emotional eating much more than others. If you feel that you might be an emotional eater, you are not alone. Experts agree that as much as **75% of overeating may be caused by emotions.**[8]

Many people, particularly those who've struggled on and off with dieting most of their lives, have disconnected from their bodies, learning to ignore signs of hunger and the cues that signal fullness, or satiation. Without mindfulness - awareness of what you're feeling both physically and emotionally - emotional eating can become a knee-jerk reaction to the onset of uncomfortable feelings.

Get In Touch With Your Feelings

The first step in establishing a healthy relationship with food is to reconnect with your body and emotions. Understand, though, that it takes at least a month to create a new habit. And if emotional eating has been a longstanding habit of yours, you won't be able to change it overnight. Be kind and patient with yourself.

Start to notice how you feel when you reach for food. Are you using food to cope, going to the fridge when you're angry or upset? Acknowledge your feelings and take a detour. Ask yourself: **What's going on? What is this emotion I'm feeling?** Then find a different way of dealing with it.

Affirm Your Values

A recent study revealed that when women who were unhappy with their weight completed a one-time, 15-minute, writing exercise about an <u>important</u> personal issue, they went on to lose 3+ pounds over approximately 3 months... while those who wrote about an <u>unimportant</u> topic gained 3 pounds! Researchers believe that reflecting on values can serve as a buffer to the stress and uncertainty that lead to emotional eating and help in maintaining self-control in difficult situations. So pull out your food journal, set the timer, and free-flow about what's important to you. Write as though no one else will read it. Come clean with what's bugging you. Your words may surprise but enlighten you.[9]

One thing you can do if you are feeling bad - but can't identify the exact emotion - is to merely be aware of the fact that you're feeling bad. Say aloud, "I'm feeling really bad right now" and try to quantify how bad you're feeling on scale of 1 to 10.

Also, determine your "feeling bad" thresholds. For example, if your "bad" rates a 5 or higher, you may need to call a friend. A lower level may warrant you working it out on your own by going for a walk or meditating. Do something that will make you feel better, not worse.

Tips for noticing feelings and dealing with emotional eating:

1. If you have the urge to eat, notice your feelings.

2. Before you reach for food ask yourself: *Have I missed a meal? Have I eaten my snack? Am I really hungry?*

3. If you have eaten on schedule, and you determine this urge could be emotional eating, acknowledge that you may have gotten into a habit of trying to fix your troubles with food. Don't panic. You're not alone.

4. Try, for just 10 minutes, to deal with your urge differently than with food. A new alternative might be:

   • Go for a walk.

   • Breathe deeply.

   • Pray or meditate.

   • Call a friend.

   • Measure your hunger cues (see Hunger Scale on page 30 in *Chapter Five, When Can I Eat?*).

   • Write in your journal.

   • Do something good for you! Take a bath. Do your nails. Make that household repair you've been putting off. Shoot some hoops. Get a haircut. Feel good about yourself!

Our emotional states can change minute by minute or hour to hour. If you still have a craving or urge after 10 or 15 minutes, go through the process again. Many times the urge or craving will pass. If you are still really hungry, eat something that you will feel good - not guilty - about.

Is it Something More?

Cravings you can't beat can signal an *addiction* to food. There - I said it - addiction. The cravings cycle can happen with many types of addictions: food, alcohol, drugs or cigarettes.

Many studies have been done on binge eating, cravings and food addictions. Some schools of thought suggest that binge eating or cravings are physiological, while others suggest that psychological, social or environmental factors may contribute. If you find that you experience cravings or binge eating, you may want to begin by experimenting with a number of strategies for controlling physiologically related cravings.

Understanding the Physiological Factors of Food Addiction

Much of the information in the following segments on food addiction, addictive foods and abstinence is culled from studies compiled in a report issued through the Food Addiction Institute in Sarasota, Florida[10]:

- *Pleasure enhancement.* Studies conducted on humans and animals have shown that the same pleasure centers of the brain triggered by addictive substances - drugs, like heroin and cocaine, or alcohol - are also activated by certain foods, especially those high in fat or intensely sweet. Like addictive drugs, some foods can trigger feel-good brain chemicals such as dopamine. Once people experience pleasure associated with increased dopamine in the brain, whether from taking drugs or eating certain foods, they quickly feel the need to eat again.

- *Pain reduction.* Overeating, binging and food addiction to sugar and flours may be related to serotonin levels in the pain-reduction centers of the brain.

- *Additional biochemical reasons.* There are studies suggesting that people with low leptin levels can suffer from overeating of all foods. Leptin, a hormone produced by fat cells, is thought to be involved in the regulation of body fat. Some people with celiac disease may find difficulty feeling satiated and tend to overeat. For others, a deficiency in insulin could contribute to a false feeling of starving, triggering an overeating or binging episode.

Binge-triggering and Addictive Foods

Below is a list of offending foods and situations that can trigger cravings and binge eating or lead to addiction:

- *Intensely sweet foods.* In some studies, intensely sweet foods surpassed cocaine as a desired reward for laboratory animals. And results were not limited to foods containing refined sugars. Intensely sweet foods made with artificial sweeteners prompted similar results!

- *High-fat foods.* While it's widely known and accepted that ingesting high levels of fat is not healthful, research conducted at Rockefeller University in 2009 revealed a double whammy: Overconsumption of fats activates certain parts of the brain to further stimulate the desire for and intake of fat. Yes, over-consuming fats can make you crave more fats. Gram for gram, fat has more than twice as many calories as protein and carbohydrate. That's why we sometimes reach for fattier foods when we're really hungry. Our body knows we'll feel fuller faster.

- *Refined foods.* A study conducted in 2009 showed that some obese adults who regularly overeat refined foods experience significant and frequent physical craving for those refined foods that prompt binging episodes.

- *Photos of offending foods.* There is evidence that pictures of the foods people binged on can trigger strong, difficult-to-overcome cravings.

- *Other known offenders.* Caffeine (found in coffee, cola, energy drinks and chocolate, to name a few items), wheat (can be found in everything from breads to soups to deli meats to ice cream –

check labels!) and salt also top the list of offending foods for many people.

Abstinence: A Strategy for Breaking the Binge Cycle

Research conducted on self-assessed food addicts in Overeaters Anonymous found that many were successful losing weight by dealing first with physical craving, then completely eliminating foods that prompted cravings and binges. Going cold turkey, though, can be difficult. If you decide on this route, I suggest having substitutes in mind and on hand to satisfy cravings that may arise.

Have a sweet tooth? Keep fresh fruits and berries on hand, and find a frozen yogurt or sorbet that is fruit only. *Have a hankering for something crunchy?* Keep crudités and/or baked whole-grain chips on hand instead of reaching for those wicked potato chips. *Is chocolate your best friend?* I like keeping unsweetened chocolate almond milk on hand to blend with frozen bananas for a chocolate-y smoothie.

As Ben Franklin once said, "If you fail to plan, you plan to fail."

When to Seek Help

If you continue to experience an ongoing, vicious cycle of uncontrolled eating, you might need to speak to *a doctor or psychologist who specializes in emotional eating disorders.* A specialized doctor can determine if you suffer from emotional eating, food addiction or binge-eating disorder (BED) and what steps to take toward healing. Treatment for binge-eating disorders spans psychotherapy, antidepressants, medically supervised weight-loss programs, and self-help strategies (books, dvds, mobile apps, support groups).

Symptoms of BED as published by the American Psychiatric Association:

- Recurrent episodes of binge eating, including eating abnormally large amounts of food and feeling a lack of control over eating

- Binge-eating episodes that have three or more of these factors: eating quickly; eating until uncomfortably full; eating a lot of food when you're not hungry; eating alone out of embarrassment; feeling depressed, guilty or disgusted after eating

- Concern about your binge eating

- Binge eating at least twice a week for at least six months

- Binge eating that's not associated with purging (self-induced vomiting)

You Are So Not Alone: Eating Disorder Statistics[11]

- Almost 50% of people with eating disorders meet the criteria for depression.[12]

- Only 1 in 10 men and women with eating disorders receive treatment. Only 35% of people that receive treatment go to a facility specializing in eating disorders.[13]

- Up to 24 million people of all ages and genders suffer from an eating disorder (anorexia, bulimia and binge-eating disorder) in the U.S.[14]

- An estimated 2 to 5 percent of Americans experience binge-eating disorder in a 6-month period.[15]

- Eating disorders have the highest mortality rate of any mental illness.[16]

- 86% of those with eating disorders report onset by age 20; 43% report onset between the ages of 16 and 20.[17]

- The body type portrayed in advertising as the ideal is possessed naturally by only 5% of American females.[18]

- 47% of girls in 5th-12th grade reported wanting to lose weight because of magazine pictures.[19]

- 69% of girls in 5th-12th grade reported that magazine pictures influenced their idea of a perfect body shape.[20]

As you can see, I've likely written more on this topic than most diet books do. But in my experience, I've found that the emotional aspect of eating is terribly underrated. You can be diligent with your food intake and journaling, and perform like an athlete at the gym. But if you do not acknowledge, assess, and deal with any underlying emotional issues that contribute to an unhealthy weight, the weight will come back. I guarantee it. If any of the statistics above feel very familiar, *please*, please, please be sure to address these issues so that your weight-loss journey (and your life) can change for the better.

Chapter Five
When Can I Eat?

Eat More. More *Often*, That Is!

Eating less or skipping meals may seem like a good strategy when you're counting calories and trying to lose weight. But in fact, there are huge benefits to eating multiple small meals and snacks throughout the day. *Biggest Loser* contestants and my private clients who are significantly overweight are often surprised to learn that one of the reasons they've *gained* so much weight is because they've been consistently *skipping* meals!

This plan has you eating 5-6 times a day, broken down into 3 meals and 2-3 snacks daily. This pattern is designed to help regulate blood sugar (if you are a type 1 diabetic, please consult your doctor or a registered dietitian), curb cravings, regulate blood pressure, and provide strength and endurance for physical activities. (See *Blood Sugar Tolerance Biomarkers* and *Blood Pressure Biomarkers, Appendix 3, page* 145.)

While it seems counterintuitive to meal-skippers that they should add a meal (or two) to their weight-loss regimen, there's a whole lot of research indicating that eating healthful, low-calorie (but high-quality) meals and snacks at regular intervals throughout the day promotes weight *loss*.

Mom Was Right! Breakfast Is the Most Important Meal of the Day!

Mornings can be a busy time. But starting each day with a nutritious meal will not only help you avoid mid-morning hunger and overeating at lunch, it can also lower your risk of disease. Consider these facts:

Studies show that eating breakfast lowers levels of that insidious stress hormone, cortisol. Cortisol makes us crave sweet starchy foods then directs our bodies to store fat around the waistline and also makes cells resistant to insulin, increasing the risk of type 2 diabetes and heart disease.

- *Eating a <u>protein-rich</u> meal <u>early in the day</u> keeps you from overeating throughout the day.* Lean protein helps balance the rise in blood sugar caused by carbohydrates, delays stomach emptying, and makes you feel full longer than carbs alone, staving off hunger. Go Pro!

- *Eating breakfast daily is a habit of successful weight losers.* According to the National Weight Control Registry (a group tracking over 10,000 individuals to learn how people lose weight and keep it off), nearly 80% of "successful" losers – those that have maintained a minimum 30-pound weight loss for at least one year – report eating breakfast *every day.* (They also maintain high-quality, low-calorie diets and exercise regularly, but we'll get to that!)

- *Skipping meals wreaks havoc on blood sugar levels.* The National Institute on Aging found that people who fasted during the day and consumed all of their calories in one nightly meal exhibited unhealthy changes in metabolism, on par with harmful blood sugar levels observed in diabetics. Conversely, blood sugar levels remained healthy in those who didn't skip meals even though they consumed the same number of daily calories as the one-meal eaters.

Even if you're not watching your weight, there are additional benefits to eating several small meals throughout the day. Eating regular small portions and healthy snacks will:

- *Help you recognize and listen to hunger and satiety cues* – signals that let us know when we need to eat and when to stop.

- *Prevent you from becoming famished.* It's when we're "starving" that we're most likely to reach for unhealthful foods and overeat.
- *Keep you energized* for physical activities.
- *Counter impulse eating* by developing regular eating patterns.

Quantifying Hunger

It's important to stay tuned in to your body's subtle hunger and satiety cues so that you're eating when necessary and know when to stop. Below is a sample of a hunger scale from my friend and colleague Lisa Sasson, MS, RD, a clinical professor of nutrition at NYU. The goal is to eat when you have the first stirrings of hunger (Level 4) and stop when you are comfortably full (Level 6). By remaining within this zone, you'll moderate your food intake and avoid both crashes and binges.

Hunger Scale

1 - Hungry, starving, dizzy, irritable
2 - Very hungry, unable to concentrate
3 - Hungry, ready to eat
4 - Beginning signals of hunger

Neutral 5 - Comfortable, neither hungry nor full

6 - Comfortably full, satisfied
7 - Very full, feel as if you have overeaten
8 - Uncomfortably full, feel stuffed
9 - Very uncomfortably full, need to loosen pants
10 - Full, stuffed, feel sick

Track your hunger level before and your satiety level after eating, and add readings to your food journal. You may recognize patterns. For example, you may find that you regularly delay eating until you're irritable (Level 1), at which point you gulp down a meal and don't realize you've overeaten. By noticing your tendencies and the cues, you can make better choices.

Divvying up Daily Calories

In *Chapter Two, How Many Calories Do I Need?*, you calculated your calorie budget. Record this number in the chart on page 167. Now that you understand the importance of eating at regular intervals, the next step is to divide your calories among daily meals and snacks.

Step 1. To determine how much you should spend on each of your three meals and 2-3 snacks each day, divide your daily calorie budget by four. Record this number in the chart on page 167 for breakfast, lunch and dinner calories. The example below uses a calorie budget of 1,200 per day (yours may be more or less, see the chart below).

Total daily calorie budget: 1,200

For each meal-breakfast, lunch and dinner-you're allotted 300 calories. So for three meals, you'd use up 900 calories, or three-fourths of your daily budget.

Step 2: Now divide the remaining one-quarter of your total calorie budget - in this example, 300 calories - by two. Record this number in the chart on page 167 for your snack calories. The calculation for grams of protein per day and grams of protein per meal and snack is found on page 41 of Chapter Six What Can I Eat?

Your two daily snacks should consist of 150 calories each.

Staying satisfied throughout the day is critical to overall success, so use this formula only as a starting point. Notice when you are feeling hungry or satiated (note it in your food journal) and adjust portions accordingly.

When Small Meals Don't Satisfy

I will never forget a *Biggest Loser* contestant who would frequent inexpensive buffets so that he could fill up on food with his small budget. As he was finishing one meal at a buffet, he was already thinking about his next meal.

Some people need that physical feeling of fullness. If this is your situation, divvy up your daily calories differently and experiment with one bigger meal. Or one big snack in the afternoon, rather than 2-3 during the day. Does this help you feel more satisfied? Write your feelings and thoughts in your journal.

Don't Forget Fluids – But Don't Drink Your Calories!

Water intake can have a positive impact on weight management. Not only can the volume of a glass of water in your belly help to make you feel full (generally speaking, it's said that water "falls through the cracks"), but *sometimes the sensation of hunger is confused with thirst.* And fluids are important for bringing nutrients and oxygen to your cells and carrying toxins away.

- *Take in plenty of fluid* during waking hours, primarily water and tea.

- *Aim for 8 to 12 glasses* of water each day.

- *Substitute antioxidant-rich green tea.* Green tea is a good source of the antioxidant EGCG, which has a mild metabolism-boosting effect. Four cups of green tea can kick up your metabolism by 80 calories, according to an article in <u>The American Journal of Clinical Nutrition</u>.[21]

- *Drink other good fluids*: calcium-rich, organic, fat-free or low-fat milk; or an occasional cup of coffee.

- *Drink a glass of water in lieu of a snack,* and you may find that you don't need to nibble.

- *Add herbs* like mint or basil or slices of citrus fruits or cucumber to infuse water with refreshing taste.

- *Yes, wine is a "fluid"* – more about that in *Chapter Six, What Can I Eat?, page 35.*

Hydrating a Workout

Consume 8 ounces of water every 20 minutes when exercising, and have 2 8-ounce glasses afterward to restore fluids. If you plan to exercise for more than an hour, increase water intake before you work out, hydrate well during exercise, then replenish your body with plenty of fluids after the event.

Write Down or Think About Your Difficult Times of Day

What are your most difficult times of day cravings-wise? What are your triggers and what foods or activities help? Be sure to plan for this with snacks, meals or activities that can satiate, occupy or distract you. Write notes in your journal on what worked.

Timing Dinner

The time that you eat dinner is not as important as how close it is to your bedtime. Eating dinner 2-3 hours or more before bedtime may help with several common issues:

- *Curb reflux (heartburn)*: Your stomach needs some time to empty before reclining. When your stomach is too full and you lie down, you may experience heartburn.

- *Aid digestion*: 2-3 hours (without snacking) before bed allows for digestion time. And you might wake up the next morning feeling a bit hungry - which is a good thing! You'll be less likely to skip breakfast.

- *Sleep better*: If you eat dinner at 5 or 6 p.m., however, and don't go to bed until 11 p.m. or later, be sure to eat a 150-calorie snack that includes carbs and lean protein 2-3 hours before bedtime.

No matter how often you eat, the trick is to choose *wisely*, whether it's your healthful breakfast, midmorning coffee break or afternoon pick-me-up. Make breakfast an opportunity to start your day off right and feed your body with nutritious options at regular intervals during the day. More on this in *Chapter Six, What Can I Eat?*

Chapter Six
What Can I Eat?

Choosing Quality Calories

When it comes to calories, quality is more important than quantity. That's right, calorie counters. Many of my overweight clients, including *The Biggest Loser* contestants, have a long history of eating and drinking too much of the *wrong* types of foods and too little of the *right* kind.

Not planning our daily meals and snacks can result in bad habits: skipping meals, getting really hungry, making bad in-the-moment food choices, grabbing quick (processed) food on the fly, and not paying attention to what or how much you're eating in a day. In most cases, grabbing food on the go, with no thought or planning, results in consumption of high-quantity empty calories – foods with little or no nutritive value.

Choosing the wrong foods, and eating too much of these foods, not only increases your odds of gaining weight and getting sick – with everything from a cold to diabetes or heart disease - but eating empty-calorie foods will also leave you feeling depleted of energy and satisfaction in the long run.

Stay away from these harmful foods and bad habits:

- *Too much red meat* (if you love red meat, have it once or twice a week and stick to **USDA** Choice or **USDA** Select grades, which are leaner cuts)
- *Fast food, processed food*
- *Foods loaded with cholesterol, salt and sugar*
- *Sodas and sugary drinks*

- *Not enough fresh fruits and vegetables*
- *Minimal fiber and antioxidants*
- *Skipped meals and eating on the run*
- *Drinking - rather than eating - calories!*

Juices, Lattes and Cocktails... Oh My!

Sugary sodas, sweetened (and unsweetened) juices, cocktails, and drive-thru drinks - including your morning latte - all have calories... in some cases, *lots* of calories. If you're trying to lose weight, these "hidden" calories might mean the difference between reaching your goal and carrying around that extra 5 or 10 (or more!) pounds you can't seem to drop. Note how many calories you're drinking each day and write it in your food journal. Then opt for non-caloric alternatives like flavored water or green tea.

Lose the Booze

If you enjoy alcohol (I do!), passing on that nightly glass (or three!) of wine could help you lose weight more quickly than you expect. But not for the reason you think. While pure alcohol contains about 7 calories per gram - which makes it nearly twice as caloric as carbohydrates or protein (both contain about 4 calories per gram) and just shy of the 9 calories per gram that fat delivers - alcohol presents additional challenges to weight loss.

Your body burns alcohol calories first, before fat, carbs or protein. That means it slows down the burning of fat. Those are the scientific facts. But a more powerful fact is that a little (or not so little) drink here and there helps you to lose inhibitions and willpower. So if you want to lose weight or reduce excess body fat, keep your libations to a minimum. Aim for one drink a day at most, and don't have it within a few hours of bedtime, or it may disrupt your sleep, too.

Right Foods

So which foods comprise quality calories? Foods that are loaded with nutrients, fiber and antioxidants, lots of water, very little bad fat (cholesterol, trans fat and saturated fat), and very little added sugar, of course!

Right foods can be found in all food groups: carbohydrates, proteins and fats. General strategies for selecting right foods:

- *Load up!* Include veggies in your breakfast, salads, sandwiches and sides. Lots of water + lots of volume = filling
- *Skip fruit juices.* Add fresh fruit to yogurt or smoothies. Eat your calories!
- *One word: Quinoa!* (pronounced KEEN-wah). Learn to love it! It's a superfood - both a grain *and* a protein!
- *Go lean.* Eat lean cuts of meat and poultry. Lose the fatty meat and high-fat dairy.
- *Eat veggie proteins.* Beans and legumes. Lentils rock!
- *Go fish.* Increase fish intake to several times a week.
- *Choose whole grains over refined "white" grains.*

Every "diet" has its own ratio of macronutrients - carbs, protein and good fats. This is the ratio I recommend to my clients and to *The Biggest Loser* cast, because it works!

- 45% of calories from carbohydrates
- 30% of calories from lean protein
- 25% of calories from good fats

Carbohydrates - 45% of Daily Calories

Refined carbohydrates - like white flour and macaroni - and the notorious popularity of low-carb and gluten-free diets have given carbs a bad name. It's true, overconsumption of the nearly empty calories in refined carbs can cause weight gain and even metabolic disorders. But your body relies on stored carbohydrates - called glycogen - to provide energy; without it, your body burns stored fat, initiating a process called ketosis, which can stress kidneys and liver. Healthy carbs are at the core of my plan:

- Aim for a minimum of 4 cups of non-starchy vegetables and fresh (not dried) fruits daily, weighted more heavily toward vegetables than fruit.

- Emphasize fresh produce and legumes, minimize grains and cereals.

- Eat grains in moderation, choosing whole grains with high fiber content.

Vegetables, the Cornerstone of a Healthy Diet

You may subscribe to the popular misconception that vegetables (without butter and cheese!) aren't filling, but nothing could be further from the truth! Most vegetables have a high water content, delivering satisfying bulk with just a few calories. Vegetables are also loaded with fiber, making you feel fuller while helping lower your risk of diabetes and heart disease.

To get a full 4 cups of veggies into your daily diet, try these strategies:
- *Go green... wisely.* In an ideal world, we'd all eat organic produce all the time, but organic tends to be more expensive than conventionally grown fruits and vegetables. If you're on a budget, focus your organic purchases on thin-skinned fruit and veggies vulnerable to pesticide exposure - peaches and apricots, cherries and bell peppers, celery and spinach.

- *One a day.* Try to eat at least one raw vegetable each day.

- *Mix 'em up.* Eat a vegetable salad most days of the week.

- *Keep veggies on hand.* Keep cut vegetables in your fridge for easy snacking.

- *Experiment!* During spring and summer, dozens of different vegetables are in season.

- *Eat what you like.* Sounds obvious, but if you hate Brussels sprouts, forcing them down will not endear vegetables to you!

- *Fire 'em up!* Roasting, puréeing or grilling fresh vegetables unlocks new flavor profiles for even the most familiar veggies. Herbs and spices can round out a rich taste experience.

- *Make veggies the main course.* Place flavorful vegetables front and center on lunch and dinner plates, accompanied by sides of protein and whole grains. Hello, Meatless Mondays.

- *Consider frozen.* Typically, vegetables are frozen immediately after harvest, retaining nutrients and vitamins. Opt for versions without added salt or sugar.

Fruits - Powerhouses of Antioxidants

Most of us need no convincing to reach for fruit. Whole fruits are excellent sources of anti-aging nutrients. Oftentimes, the nutrients and vitamins are found in the pigments of fruits (and veggies), so go for color!

Pomegranates are the most concentrated source of antioxidants, while *blueberries* contain compounds that not only prevent loss of age-related impairments of memory and motor coordination, but that also may help reverse the process. *Berries* contain antioxidants with triple the power of vitamin C, known to block cancer-causing cell damage and the effects of many age-related diseases. *Citrus fruits* are loaded with antioxidants offering protection against chronic conditions that develop over a lifetime such as heart disease, diabetes and high blood pressure.

Some guidelines for incorporating fruit into your daily plan:

- *One a day.* Enjoy at least one raw fruit each day.

- *Opt for fresh fruit whenever possible.* Dried fruits are more concentrated in sugar and calories than raw fruit. And they're not as filling.

- *Choose whole fruit rather than juices.* Juice contains more sugar and less fiber than whole fruit and isn't as filling as the real deal.

- *Do it for dessert.* Substitute a beautifully presented tropical fruit - like mango or kiwi - for dessert!

- *Frozen fruit without added syrup or sugar* is OK, too.

- *Don't overdo it!* Some fruits have a relatively high sugar content. Watch your portion sizes.

Whole Grains - Unsung Hero

Whole grains are nutritious because, unlike refined grains, all parts of the plant, including the fiber-rich outer layer (the bran) and the vitamin-rich seed (the germ), have been left intact. Whole grains deliver powerful nutrients and antioxidants that bolster immunity, help prevent cancer and heart disease, and slow aging. As with most things, moderation is key.

Good whole-grain selections to incorporate into your meals are:

√ Barley

√ Bulgur

√ Oats (gluten-free options available; see *Resources, page* 152)

√ Quinoa (is gluten-free)

√ Polenta (is gluten-free)

√ Brown rice (is gluten-free)

√ Wild rice (is gluten-free)

Did you know? Quinoa is a complete protein

Amino acids are the building blocks of protein, and they fall into two categories: essential amino acids, which your body doesn't produce on its own, and nonessential amino acids, which your body can make on its own. Because we humans can't make essential amino acids on our own, we need to consume an adequate amount of all of them (there are nine).

Does that sound like a bunch of mumbo-jumbo? It's not. Here's why: A source of protein that contains all nine essential amino acids in correct proportions for supporting important functions in your body is called a complete protein. And — here's the really super news — quinoa is one of the few nonmeat and nondairy foods that contains all nine essential amino acids! In other words, quinoa is a complete protein source.

Quinoa is a great food choice for anyone, especially those following a vegan or gluten-free diet. Because quinoa contains all the essential amino acids and is high in protein, it's a scrumptious food that helps build muscle tissue. There's a reason Incan warriors ate quinoa before going into battle. It provides overall good nutrition and energy and is a complete protein that's perfect for everyone.[22]

Packaged Grains: Proceed with Caution

- *Read labels.* A necessity for bread and grain products.

- *"Enriched" - not so much!* Translation: contains white flour, likely low in fiber and nutrition, and typically high in empty calories.

- *Breads.* Choose those with at least 2 grams of fiber per serving. The first ingredient listed should be whole wheat or whole grain.

- *Wheat flour.* Guess what? Wheat flour is frequently enriched white flour with *very little* whole wheat added. Look for the word "whole" on labels.

- *Beware of breakfast cereals.* Most are highly processed and have lots of added sugar. Select varieties with less than 5 grams of sugar and at least 5 grams of fiber per serving.

- *Avoid low-carb or no-carb bread products.* They are often full of processed ingredients and chemicals

- *Ask for whole grain.* Always.

Protein - 30% of Daily Calories

Protein is found throughout your entire body - in every cell, tissue and organ - and your body is constantly using and replacing proteins. Just a few of the vital functions proteins perform:

- *Protein builds and repairs tissues including muscles, hair, skin and blood vessels.* Protein also helps your muscles recover from tough workouts.

- *Protein-rich foods are a good source of essential nutrients* - calcium, iron, selenium and zinc - that help build strong bones, reduce cancer risk and protect your immune system.

- *Eating a combination of protein and carbohydrates helps slow the release of sugars into your bloodstream,* preventing blood sugar spikes. This combo also helps you feel fuller.

For these reasons, roughly 30% of your daily calories should come from protein. Focus on high-quality protein - including plant sources - to create entrees, side dishes and snacks that are healthful *and* satisfying.

How much protein do you need in a day? Some people may require more based on body size, lean body mass and activity level.

To calculate your daily protein requirements, multiple your daily calorie budget times 30%. eg 1200 calories x .3 = 360 or 360 protein calories per day.

There are four calories in a gram of protein. To calculate the number of grams of protein per day, divide your calories of protein by four. eg 360 protein calories /4 = 90 grams of protein per day.

Divide the number of protein grams per day by four to calculate the number of protein grams per meal. 90/4 = 22.5 grams protein per meal. Record this number in the chart on page 167.

Divide the number of protein grams per meal by two to calculate the number of protein grams per snack eg 22.5 = 11.25 or approximately 11 protein grams per snack. Record this number in the chart on page 167.

Here is an example of the complete calculation in summary using a 1200 calories per day budget:

Daily Calorie Budget = 1200 Calories

Daily Protein Calories = 1200 x .3 = 360 Protein Calories

Daily Protein Grams = 360/4 = 90 Grams of Protein

Daily Protein Grams Per Meal = 90/4 = 22.5 or ~ 23 Grams Protein Per Meal

Record this number in the chart on page 167.

Daily Protein Grams Per Snack = 22.5/2 = 11.25 Grams Protein Per Snack

Record this number in the chart on page 167

Remember, you will be eating 3 meals and 2 snacks per day.

Daily Calorie Budget	1200
Calories per meal	300
Calories per snack	150
Protein calories per day	360
Protein grams per meal	23
Protein grams per snack	11

Daily Calorie Budget	1500
Calories per meal	375
Calories per snack	188
Protein calories per day	450
Protein grams per meal	28
Protein grams per snack	14

Daily Calorie Budget	1800
Calories per meal	450
Calories per snack	225
Protein calories per day	540
Protein grams per meal	34
Protein grams per snack	17

Protein is vital to good health and should play an important role in every meal and snack. To ensure that you get enough healthy protein:

- *Choose a variety* of animal or vegetable proteins each day.

- *Include protein with every meal and every snack.* Your body uses it throughout the day.

- *Choose fish several times a week.* Fish is an excellent source of protein, omega-3 fatty acids, vitamin E and selenium.

- *Limit lean red meat consumption* to once or twice a week. Red meat tends to be higher in saturated fat and cholesterol, so be sure to choose lean cuts.

- *Avoid processed meats*: deli meats, hot dogs and sausage. They're generally high in fat and calories and may also contain carcinogenic sodium nitrites.

Let's take a closer look at various protein sources.

Animal protein

Meat

- *Choose lean cuts* such as pork tenderloin and beef round, chuck, sirloin or tenderloin.

- *Avoid heavily marbled* meat, remove visible fat.

- *Use ground meat that is at least 95% lean.*

- *USDA Choice or USDA Select* grades of beef typically have lower fat content.

- *Grass-fed beef* has a significantly lower fat content than grain fed. And grass-fed beef is rich in omega-3s, the polyunsaturated "good" fatty acids that are essential nutrients for healthy bodies. Since our bodies can't make omega-3s, we need to eat foods that contain them.

Poultry

- *Skinless chicken or turkey breast* meat is leanest.

- *Ask for white meat* when purchasing ground chicken or turkey.

Seafood

- *Salmon, sardines (water-packed), herring, mackerel, trout, anchovies and tuna* are favored selections, as they are rich in omega-3 fatty acids.

- *Choose wild* when you have the option.

Dairy

In addition to supplying protein, dairy is a good source of vitamin D and calcium, both of which - when consumed in adequate amounts - have proven to help reduce the risk of certain cancers. The key is choosing wisely – opt for low-fat or fat-free products to reduce intake of saturated fat. Aim for 2 servings per day, and select according to the following guidelines:

- **Go slim.** Fat-free milk is always your best option. If you want something richer in your morning coffee, keep 1% milk on hand.

- **Go live.** Many yogurts contain probiotics – referred to as "live cultures" on the label. These healthy bacteria help you digest food better and can boost your immune system.

- **Go light on cheese.** Choose low-fat or reduced-fat mozzarella, string cheese and feta – and definitely skip the Brie. Rule of thumb; harder cheeses generally have less fat, and calories.

- **Go white(s).** Egg whites are an excellent fat-free source of protein. And a yolk or two is fine, but just remember that yolks have more fat and calories. You can also get an extra nutrient boost from yolks laid by chickens fed a diet rich in omega-3 fatty acids.

- **Go Greek.** Greek-style yogurt packs a protein wallop of *two times* more protein than other yogurts. Choose unsweetened, low-fat or fat-free.

Vegetarian Protein

Excellent sources of vegetarian protein include beans and legumes and traditional soy foods such as tofu and edamame. Legumes are loaded with protein, making them a good alternative to meat. A half cup of cooked black beans has 215 calories and less than 1 gram of fat, but 8 grams of protein! By comparison, a 3-ounce serving of broiled lean sirloin has 158 calories and 26 grams of protein... but a whopping 6 grams of fat, almost one-half of which is unhealthy saturated fat.

Only soybeans are considered a "complete" protein – meaning they contain all nine amino acids essential to building protein in the body. Other beans, along with nuts and seeds, are "incomplete" proteins, meaning they lack one or more of those amino acids. The good news is that whole grains make up for what legumes lack, and together they make a complete protein factory and a great flavor combination.

Pistachio Principle[1]

Behavioral eating expert James Painter, Ph.D., R.D. found that eating pistachios may help individuals consume fewer calories without consciously restricting their calories, which he calls the "Pistachio Principle."

He has conducted two separate studies that speak to this point:

- One study found the pistachio shell, which is left behind after snacking on the nut, actually provides a visual cue to how much you've eaten. Unlike other common snacks and nuts that leave no evidence behind, the empty pistachio shell seems to help regulate the desire to overeat.

- Findings from Dr. Painter's second study suggest that physically removing the shell from the pistachio actually slows down the eating process, which helps you to manage how many you eat without compromising fullness.

Good Fats - 25% of Daily Calories

Fat gets its bad rep because it is high in calories and because some fats - such as saturated fats found in meat and whole-milk dairy products and trans fats found in many processed and fried foods - can increase artery-blocking **LDL** ("bad") cholesterol. Elevated **LDL** levels can contribute to heart disease and high blood pressure.

Although fat has long been the bad boy of the weight-loss industry, it's important to understand that good fats go hand in hand with a healthy diet. Here's why: Some of the unsaturated fats found in vegetable and seed oils deliver health benefits, lowering **LDL** counts and boosting levels of **HDL** ("good" cholesterol) that helps clear **LDL** from the bloodstream.

---

[1]Appetite   Volume 57, Issue 2, October 2011, Pages 418–420
"The effect of pistachio shells as a visual cue in reducing caloric consumption"
K. Kennedy-Hagan, J.E. Painter, C. Honselman, A. Halvorson, K. Rhodes, K. Skwir

As with all calorie-dense foods, moderation is key. Fat should account for no more than 25% of your daily caloric intake. A good percentage of your daily fat calories will be spent on healthful fats hidden in proteins and carbohydrates, and you will have a small number of fat calories left over each day for extras such as nuts and seeds, and healthful oils. There are two main categories of healthful oils:

- Vegetable oils are extracted from plant matter: olive oil. Seed oils are a subset of vegetable oils made from pressed plant seeds delivering highly concentrated nutrients and flavors in small doses: flaxseed oil, grapeseed oil, sesame oil.

- Nut oils are a good source of beneficial fats but tend to be pricier: walnut oil, almond oil.

For information on cooking with oils, see *Chapter Nine, Cooking Tools and Techniques*, and *Appendix 1*.

Snacking Promotes Weight LOSS!

That's right. Snacking is integral to a healthy diet. So, what do I mean by that? It does not mean that you can rip into a bag of chips every time you get the urge. It *does* mean that you should keep lots of healthful snacks available, so when you open the refrigerator you can only make the right choices.

A healthful snack should be comprised of both protein and carbohydrate and hover at around 150 calories, give or take, depending on your calorie budget (more on page 31).

A good strategy for ensuring healthful snacking is keeping enough snack-ready fresh vegetables and proteins on hand to keep you satiated (or feeling full) throughout the day.

- *Carrots.* Buy baby carrots and keep them handy for snacking, or just slice some regular-sized carrots into spears. In an airtight container or plastic bag, they'll stay fresh for up to two weeks. An entire cup of carrots has just 52 calories (plus several days' worth of vitamin A). Serve them with a high-protein dip like hummus and you have the perfect snack.

- *Veggies for the fridge.* Broccoli, cauliflower, cucumbers, peppers, summer squash, whole green beans or wax beans will stay fresh for at least 3-5 days in an airtight container or bag.

- *Fruits* intended to ripen after picking (tomatoes included) should not be refrigerated at all, and are lovely to keep out in the open in a bowl. Consider keeping whole apples, pears, peaches and nectarines within arm's reach at home or your office for between-meal snacks.

- *Low- or reduced-fat mozzarella, cheddar or other cheese sticks* provide quick and easy protein. Pair it with an apple for a satisfying snack.

These are just the tip of the iceberg. For more snack options, see Appendix 1.

What if You're Vegan?

Most people eat plenty of protein on a daily basis. But if you follow a strict vegan diet, you may need to focus a bit more on making sure you get the daily protein you need. Include high-protein foods like lentils, beans, whole grains and quinoa and you should have no problem meeting your protein goal. The following is a list of some high-protein foods for vegetarians:

- Tempeh
- Tofu
- Soybeans
- Beans (black, kidney, chickpeas, pinto)
- Quinoa (see *Quinoa: A complete protein, page 40*)
- Peas
- Soy milk

Vegetarians, especially vegans, are at risk for vitamin B-12 deficiency. After you become a true vegetarian, the body stores of vitamin B-12 can become depleted over a couple of years' time if you're not supplementing or eating products that are B-12 fortified (and there are many of them). This vitamin is naturally found in liver, beef, seafood, cheese, eggs and whole cow's milk. If you are a vegan, talk with your doctor or health care provider to find out if or how you should supplement this vitamin.

What if You're Gluten Free?

Gluten is a protein found in wheat, rye and barley (and most oats through cross-contamination). If you are banishing gluten from your diet, quinoa - a complete protein - is a great choice. Other good options: corn (corn tortillas, etc.), gluten-free oats and rice (brown and wild are best choices).

Chapter Seven
Build and Burn -
Exercising for Weight Loss

Get Off the Couch - Just Do It!

There are many more good reasons to exercise than there are excuses not to. Exercise not only burns those pesky extra calories that add inches to your waistline, but exercise that builds and maintains muscle also kicks up your metabolism, helping your body burn more calories 24/7.

Beyond weight loss, the additional benefits of exercise are hard to ignore. Did I mention that strengthening your muscles also strengthens your bones? Exercise can alter your mood, reduce stress, boost energy, help fight disease, promote sleep ... and even improve your sex life! Hubba hubba!

For most of us, weight creep - that slow, insidious weight gain, particularly around the midsection - is generally due to a combination of decreased physical activity and exercise, hard-to-avoid bouts of stress and its ugly partner cortisol, loss of muscle mass, and eating too many calories.

Exercise: A Necessity as We Age

Maintaining muscle mass to fend off weight gain grows increasingly difficult with age, however. At around 30 years old, we all begin to experience the onset of muscle mass decline, dwindling some 3% to 8% each decade. At 60, these losses accelerate even more quickly. Your nervous system becomes less efficient at prompting muscles to move, while fat and connective tissue invade your muscles, leaving less muscle to move your body.

So even if your body weight has stayed the same over time, its composition likely has not. Without exercise, your muscles shrink and fat levels increase). Internally, this extra fat increases your risk of diabetes, stroke and some cancers. Externally, your body shape changes, meaning bigger jeans and fewer fitted tops.

But the consequences are far more serious than a change in appearance. Your muscle mass and bone strength determine how healthy and active you'll remain for the rest of your life. With the most recent available data reporting U.S. life expectancy hovering between 78-79 years old[23], there's ample incentive to stay healthy, and strong, beyond 60. (See *Bone Density Biomarkers, Appendix 3, page 145.*)

Customize Your Exercise Regimen

While aerobic exercises like running, bicycling, swimming and dancing help you burn calories, they generally don't help build much muscle. For that we all need resistance (strength) training. Your workouts should comprise a combination of resistance training and aerobic exercise that's compatible with your age and lifestyle.

Measuring Muscle vs. Fat.

A quick, easy, and cost-effective way to measure fat loss is with an ordinary tape measure. Ask a friend or family member to place a nonmetal tape measure around your waist, parallel to the floor at belly-button level. After you let out a breath, have your helper take two waist circumference readings – do additional readings if these two differ by more than one-half inch. This measurement, coupled with your baseline weight, can be an effective way to track progress. I always ask my clients to measure their waistline each week when they weigh in. If they're following my plan and the scale doesn't move, the tape measure usually does. (See Muscle vs Fat Biomarkers, Appendix 3, page 139.)

How Much is Enough?

- *Aerobic activity.* For healthy adults, the Department of Health and Human Services recommends getting at least 150 minutes a week of moderate aerobic activity - such as brisk walking or swimming - or 75 minutes a week of vigorous aerobic activity, such as running. For weight loss, particularly if you have more than a few pounds to lose, I recommend 60 minutes of aerobic activity at least 4-5 days a week. (To check your *Aerobic Biomarkers, see Appendix 3, page 143.*)

- *Resistance strength training.* Strength train at least twice a week.

Build Strength with Resistance Training

So the goal of resistance training is to build muscle mass and muscle strength. But what, exactly, is resistance training?

Resistance training is any activity that requires your muscles to push against a form of resistance - weights, elastic exercise bands, or even your own body weight - to build muscle strength.

Studies observing athletes who have been running all their lives found that, though they're leaner and have lower risk of chronic diseases, without supplemental strength training their strength is similar to sedentary people of the same age. "The only type of exercise that prevents [muscle loss] is resistance exercise," says William Evans, Ph.D., adjunct professor in the geriatrics program at the Duke University Medical Center who has studied how older people can address muscle decline. (To check your *Strength Biomarkers, see Appendix 3, page 141.*)

It's beyond the scope of this book to tell you everything you need to know about strength training, but here are some tips and guidelines:

- *Talk with your doctor.* Lifting weights may not be appropriate for everyone; you may need to find a low-stress alternative.

- *Hire a trainer* – even for only one session – to show you how to safely execute resistance techniques and use equipment. A certified personal trainer can help you design a program, teach you how to do exercise, and observe your form to ensure that it's correct. To find a qualified trainer near you, try **IDEA Health & Fitness Association** (ideafit.com/find-personal-trainer)

- *Lift or resist weight that is heavy enough to build muscle.* Evans recommends incorporating at least 60% (up to 80%) of the weight <u>you can lift one time</u>. The weight you use should tire you out within 8 to 12 repetitions. For example, if you can curl a 30-pound dumbbell once, you should aim for curling a 20-pound dumbbell up to 12 times. Curling a 10-pound dumbbell 20 times, by contrast, won't build your muscle strength.

- *Work opposing muscles proportionally.* That means working muscles on the front and back of your upper arms, upper back and chest, lower back and abdomen. Ignoring muscle groups can throw your body out of balance.

- *Strive for two strength-training workouts per week.*

- *Warm up 5-10 minutes before, and cool down afterward.*

- *Women, don't worry about bulking up.* If you're concerned about turning into the Incredible Hulk, don't be. Few women actually gain significant muscle mass doing strength exercises, unless they're genetically predisposed to it.

- *Your strength-training plan must be progressive.* As muscles get stronger, they adapt to lifting a certain weight. You need to add repetitions and use heavier weights (increase resistance) over time.

In as little as two months, your strength could double. It isn't simply a matter of your muscles getting bigger – your brain learns how to use your muscles more efficiently, too.

Burn, baby, burn. Calories, that is!

Running is the ultimate way to burn calories in a short period of time. It's free, doesn't require fancy equipment, and you can do it just about anywhere - rain or shine. But if you can't run because of injuries, try cycling, tap dancing, swimming or a multitude of other lower-impact aerobic exercises. Whatever you do, make sure your intensity level - how hard the activity feels to you and how hard your heart is working - is adequate for calorie burning. If you can still talk on your cellphone while you're exercising, it's **NOT** intense enough.

There are two ways to fairly accurately measure exercise intensity:

- *Your perceived exertion.* How hard does the physical activity feel to you while you're doing it? Your level of exertion may be different than that of someone who is more or less fit than you are.

Looking for a Fun Way to Burn Calories?

Make every moment - and movement - count. Few of us have two hours free each day to hit the gym. But even 15 minutes can make a difference. Watching your child's soccer game? Walk a lap around the field during halftime. Yawning through a conference call at work? Stand up and stretch. In 15 minutes, you can burn calories doing almost anything (including eating!). Calories burned in 15 minutes (based on a 150-pound person):

Kickball 125	Shuffleboard 54
Juggling 72	Grocery Shopping 63
Ice Skating 161	Ironing Clothes (standing) 41
Ballroom Dancing (slow) 63	Eating (sitting) 27
Ballroom Dancing (fast) 107	Eating (standing) 36
Tap Dancing 107	

For more ideas, check out the book The Fidget Factor, which lists dozens of ways to burn extra calories throughout the day.[24]

- *Your heart rate.* The higher your heart rate during physical activity, the higher the intensity. For greater accuracy, wear a heart rate monitor during exercise; relatively inexpensive ones are available for personal training. Please check with your health professional and/ or certified personal trainer for heart rate guidelines. Studies have shown that perceived exertion correlates well with actual heart rate. So if you think you're working hard (or not), you're probably right.[25]

Intensify It

When you fall into a comfortable exercise routine, your metabolism slacks off, so keep it interesting and supercharged. By adding intense "intervals" in your aerobic sessions, you can really burn fat and rev up your metabolism. For example, jog for 4 minutes, run fast for a one-minute interval (the fifth minute), then go back to jogging, and repeat over and over. Your body will work harder and burn more fat.

Have a Backup Plan or Change it Up

You're human. Some days you're full of enthusiasm for exercising and some days, well... you're not. For those days, have some backup options ready:

Cheryl says:

Exercising should be fun! When I feel my routine getting a bit dull, I pull out my hula hoop! Mine is a run-of-the-mill, toy store hula hoop that I've had for years (fancier, weighted versions designed for exercise are available). Not only can I work up a sweat with my hoop (in fact, according to a study sponsored by the American Council on Exercise, exercising with a weighted hoop can burn as many calories as step aerobics, brisk walking or boot camp), but hooping also always brightens my mood. I'm not sure if it's because hooping makes me feel like a carefree kid, or because it reminds me of the time when, as an adult, I won a hula hooping contest (ironically, the grand prize was a 5-pound bag of M&Ms!), but I always feel exhilarated when I'm done!

- *Shorten your normal workout.* Commit to doing 10-15 minutes of your normal workout. Chances are you'll get started and, once the endorphins start to flow, you just might complete the whole thing. If not, pat yourself on the back for doing 15 when you wanted to take a nap or eat a bag of chips instead.

- *High-intensity, shortened regimens.* High-intensity circuit training can provide health benefits in less time than traditional programs. Find one that works for you (many are on DVD) to pop into the TV on a day when time is scarce.

- *Change venues.* If you normally work out at the gym after work, go for a run at lunchtime or wake up early and run the neighbor hood. Sometimes the change of pace (pun intended!) is the breath of fresh air (again, pun intended) that can rejuvenate your routine!

- *Stress-relief programs.* On days when you're too stressed out to exercise (it happens!) opt for yoga, Pilates or tai chi for a more calming effect.

Book It

Making time *every day* for the exercise you need can be a struggle. But intense exercise is required for a healthy body and healthy mind (and sexy clothes). Book it on your calendar with the same priorities as your business or personal appointments. Remember: You don't need a huge chunk of time to meet your exercising goal:

- *Aim for 60 minutes daily*, 4-5 days - or more - a week. If you fall short of 60 a few days a week, you're still logging solid exercise time.

- *Resistance training* 2-3 days a week.

- *Do something you love*, and you'll do it rather than dread it!

- *Stay fueled.* Eat breakfast and snacks, don't skip meals and hydrate adequately.

- *Calendar it!* If it's inked, you'll be less inclined to miss.

- *Break it up.* If your schedule is super hectic, break exercise into 15-20 minute blocks.

- *Squeeze it in.* Be prepared to exercise during unforeseen lulls during the day. Have gear on hand in your car, keep dumbbells on your desk, stand when talking on the phone or watching TV, walk the dog.

- *Be social.* Make a date with a friend or co-worker. You'll be less likely to skip *and* you'll squeeze in social time. Or join a team. Team camaraderie can not only bolster your commitment to exercise, but socialization can also have a positive impact on your mood and outlook.

Fueling Your Workouts

The right timetable is variable, as there are several factors to consider: How long will you be exercising, what time of day, what kind of exercise, and what level of intensity? Experiment with quantities and timing, but try to stick to the guidelines below.

Be sure to eat breakfast. If you exercise in the morning, be sure to wake up early enough to fit in at least a small meal that includes a good source of protein.

Don't skip meals. Use timing guidelines for before/during/after exercise meals.

Pile on the protein. The recommended daily allowance for women ages 19-70+ is 46 grams of protein, for men 19-70+ it's 56 grams. I recommend a guideline of 30% of your calories to come from protein (45% from carbohydrates and 25% from fat - see *Chapter Six, What Can I Eat?, page 41*) to ensure that you have enough to support muscle maintenance and growth.

Drink 2 cups of water prior to exercising and make sure to drink during and after exercising as well.

Before Exercise

Eat a small meal or snack and hydrate with 2-3 cups of water 1-2 hours before working out. The closer it is to your exercise time, the smaller the meal/snack should be. Include carbohydrates (which will be stored in your body as glycogen – that's what your muscles use for energy) and a lean protein such as egg whites, low-fat cheese, cottage cheese, yogurt or lean meat.

During Exercise

Drink plenty of water – 1 cup every 15-20 minutes of exercise is ideal. If you plan to exercise longer than 60-90 minutes, you may benefit from an electrolyte drink (natural beverages like coconut water or sports drinks) to replace some of the electrolytes lost through sweat. These drinks contain calories, approximately 30-60 calories per cup, and a liter supplies about 60 grams of carbohydrates per hour which is what is recommended for extended activity. Bring water/drinks with you if you plan to be hiking, biking or doing anything outdoors. If you plan on being outside for many hours, bring along some food to snack on such as fresh fruit and low-fat cheese, or a sandwich made on whole-grain bread with lean protein such as sliced turkey. Take a cooler if you can, otherwise stick to nonperishable items such as trail mix, nuts or apples.

After Exercise

Hydrate, hydrate, hydrate! Drink at least 2-3 cups of water after a workout for every pound lost. Ideally, you can weigh yourself before and after a workout. For every pound lost, drink 2-3 cups of water. If you've been exercising for more than 90 minutes, drink a single serving of an electrolyte beverage (coconut water or sports drink) to restore electrolytes lost in sweat. You'll also need to replace those glycogen stores in your body by eating carbohydrates. And don't forget protein. Eating within 30 minutes of a workout is optimal for muscle-building, at most try to eat within 2 hours. And studies have shown that a ratio of 4:1 (carbs to protein) is ideal for a post-exercise snack.

Good post-exercise, glycogen-replacing snacks:

- 2 slices of whole-wheat toast with 1/2 cup of low-fat cottage cheese

- One small apple and approximately two and a half tablespoons almond butter

- One medium banana and one stick of low-fat string cheese

- 12 almonds and one medium orange

- One cup multigrain cereal with one cup nonfat milk and 1/2 cup halved strawberries

- One large whole-wheat pita with 1/4 cup hummus

Nutrient Timing: Eating After Exercise Builds a Stronger, Leaner Body
by John L. Ivy, Ph.D.

The last thing most people want to do when exercising to lose weight is eat right after an intense workout. While it may seem counterintuitive, doing exactly that – drinking a supplement or eating a small meal post-workout – can actually be extremely beneficial.

The problem. Intense exercise forces the body into a state of breakdown (catabolic state). Blood insulin levels are low and cortisol levels are high, carbohydrate stores in muscles and liver are reduced or depleted, and muscle protein breakdown is elevated. This catabolic state will continue for hours unless action is taken to shift the body into an anabolic – or recovery – state.

The science. Carbohydrate and protein ingested in the minutes after exercise help initiate a metabolic shift in the body from a state of breakdown to a state of recovery by raising blood insulin levels, lowering cortisol and other catabolic hormones, and increasing fuel availability. Just-exercised muscle is very responsive to nutrients and highly insulin sensitive. Therefore, blood glucose and amino acids are rapidly absorbed, facilitating rapid replenishment of carbohydrate stores in the muscles and liver, reduction of muscle protein breakdown and soreness, and an increase in muscle protein synthesis. Post-exercise nutrition results in a faster recovery period.

The evidence. Not convinced? Then consider this: In a recent study, participants of a 4.5-week exercise training program who received a carbohydrate/protein supplement immediately post-exercise had *twice the improvement in aerobic fitness* than participants who received a supplement with no calories. Interestingly, total daily caloric intake did not differ between the two groups, suggesting that the post-exercise supplement reduced normal food consumption later in the day. Although weight loss was the same for both groups, the participants receiving the carbohydrate/protein supplement had *better changes in body composition including greater increases in muscle mass and greater reductions in fat mass.*

The solution. A post-exercise carbohydrate/protein supplement will promote a more desirable body composition by reducing body fat while maintaining or increasing lean body mass. For intense exercise training lasting longer than 45 minutes, supplement with 0.5 grams of carbohydrate and 0.2 grams of protein per pound of body weight. For example, if you weigh 150 pounds, that would mean 7.5 grams of carbohydrate (150 x .05) and 3 grams of protein (150 x .02). If your workout is light, reduce the amount of carb and protein intake proportionally, by as much as 50%.

Many packaged products, such as low-fat chocolate milk or cereal, will have the carbohydrate and protein measurements - gram content per serving - on the container or label. If you decide to eat turkey breast on rye bread as a post-exercise snack, you may have to look up the protein and carbohydrate percentages in these foods. While there are a number of good exercise recovery supplements on the market, a couple of ordinary foods that work quite well are low-fat chocolate milk and Greek yogurt.

Timing-wise, eating as soon as possible up to 45 minutes after exercise is optimal - you'll feel better, have more energy the rest of the day, and develop a much stronger, leaner body!

John L. Ivy, Ph.D., *is professor emeritus, Department of Kinesiology and Health Education at the University of Texas at Austin. Ivy is an expert in the areas of exercise physiology, carbohydrate metabolism, exercise and diabetes, and nutrition and exercise.*

Chapter Eight
Stocking Your Kitchen the *Losing Big* Way

Fresh and Healthy

Let's take a look at the best ways to stock your kitchen with the greatest foods available to help you achieve your goals. *Buy the freshest, highest-quality foods you can afford.* Meals made with fresh, whole ingredients will likely be so much more satisfying and filling than the processed foods you previously consumed that you may find you need less food overall and can spend a little more on quality.

Tips to help you maximize your fresh-food dollar:

- *Buy seasonal and local produce.* Many items in supermarkets travel miles and miles to reach our shelves. Check store signage or ask a produce specialist where produce was grown.

- *Visit a local farmers market for fresh, just-picked produce.* Better value, better taste.

- *Shop more frequently and buy less food.* There's nothing worse than buying fresh food only to have it spoil.

- *Get to know your butcher and fishmonger.* They are a wealth of information about which cuts of meat are most tender or flavorful and which fish are in season, local or plentiful (meaning they cost less and taste better!). Plus, they are usually very happy to debone meats and fish, remove skins and offer cooking tips.

- *Grow your own.* A sunny windowsill or a few pots is plenty of room to start your own patch of basil, rosemary or thyme. If you have room outside, consider planting a few of your favorite veggies.

Ready, Set, Go Shopping!

For most of us, hunting, growing and gathering our food on a large scale just isn't feasible, so you'll need to plan for at least a weekly stop (or three) at a grocery store or supermarket.

As wonderful as many specialty or organic produce stores are, many people on a budget either can't afford to shop at these stores or very simply don't have access. Becoming accustomed to the format, layout and customer programs (such as loyalty cards) of the national supermarket, grocery and food discount chains can have its benefits, particularly if you travel and need to be able to shop anywhere.

Finding Farmers Markets

The number of farmers markets has tripled in the past 15 years. They're a great source of locally grown, fresh produce and a fun way to learn about growers and foods in your area. The USDA's searchable directory of farmers markets now includes more than 6,000 listings. It also includes listings for groceries that supply organic produce and information about Community Supported Agriculture programs (CSAs), explained in the next item on this list. search.ams.usda.gov/farmersmarkets.

General tips for navigating the supermarket:

- *Bring a list (and don't shop when you're hungry!)*. The best time to put together your shopping list is on a full stomach.

- *Join the loyalty program*. Discounts and bonuses afforded regular customers can add up to big savings at checkout.

- *Ask questions*. Typically, supermarkets will provide easy access to the butcher, fishmonger and produce staff. Many stores now have their own registered dietitians.

- *Survey store layout and start in sections with the freshest items*. Load up on produce, fish, meats and dairy (aisle locations vary from store to store... the perimeter of the store is no longer the safest place to shop!), then move to frozen, canned and packaged-goods aisles.

There are plenty of healthy pantry and freezer options in these aisles, but if you fill your cart with fresh items first, you'll be less susceptible to temptation.

- *Organic and/or fresh are best.* If buying fresh is sometimes a stretch for you, frozen foods are good, too, as they are processed quickly to preserve vitamins. Canned vegetables are better than no vegetables, but not great because many water soluble vitamins are lost (and salt is often added) in the canning process.

Perimeter Paranoia
by Leah McGrath, RD, LDN

How many times have you said or heard things like "ONLY shop the PERIMETER of the store" or "the BEST foods are in the PERIMETER of the store"? The "perimeter" reference is a tired cliché and, much like "don't eat WHITE food," needs to be taken out of dietitian-speak. If you are a consumer, the perimeter message may not be a good or accurate one to live by. Why?

1. In response to this old widespread adage, most supermarkets have changed store floor plans in recent years. Store perimeters now house cake, sausage, bacon, high-sodium lunch meats, soda, beer, wine and videos. Sure, they may also have fresh meat, seafood and produce, but if you take that "perimeter" message literally you aren't going to be making the best choices.

2. There are healthful, nutritious and economical items in the center of the store like beans, whole grains (brown rice, whole-wheat pasta), canned and jarred tomato products (good source of lycopene!), frozen fruits and vegetables.

3. The outdated "perimeter" message masks what dietitians really want to - and should - teach people: Read the Nutrition Facts label and shop for healthy options throughout the store.

4. Some people cannot or don't want to buy everything fresh. Good news! Advanced technology enables growers and manufacturers to provide economically priced, high-quality frozen fruits and vegetables that provide vitamins and minerals throughout the year.

Deciphering Food Labels

When you're shopping for healthy foods, Nutrition Facts labels can help you choose between similar products by identifying differences between calories and nutrients like fats or protein. Manufacturers are required to provide this information, and the mandatory components must appear in the order that reflects the priority of current health issues:

- Total calories
- Calories from fat
- Total fat
- Saturated fat
- Cholesterol
- Sodium
- Total carbohydrate
- Dietary fiber
- Sugars
- Protein
- Vitamin A
- Vitamin C
- Calcium
- Iron

Reading Labels

Despite the good intentions, nutrition labels can be tricky to navigate. Pay close attention to the following information:

- *Serving size*. The most important measurement to take note of is serving size because everything else on the label (calories, fat grams, etc.) is calculated based on serving size. If a serving size for a particular product is one cup, look at the calories and fat one cup represents before you decide on whether the food is a good selection for you. If you need to, cut the serving size in half (or double it).

- *Calories*. Before you record the number of calories on the label into your food journal, be sure it corresponds with your actual serving size. If the label says a serving is 1 cup and you're having 2 cups, double the calories you record in your food journal.

- *Reduced calorie* means the food contains at least 25 percent fewer calories than the regular version.

- *Low calorie* means a serving size (or designated amount) has no more than 40 calories (except sugar substitutes).

- Calorie-free means less than 5 calories for a serving size (or designated amount).

- *Protein*. High-protein foods are those that have more than 9 grams of protein per serving

- *Carbohydrate*. This number is calculated by adding grams of complex carbs + grams of fiber + grams of sugar. If the amount of total carbohydrate grams is more than double the amount of sugars, that means there are more "good carbs" in the food than bad carbs.

- *Dietary Fiber*. Fiber is found in plant foods but not in animal foods. Unless you're on a fiber-restricted diet, aim for at least 25 to 35 grams of fiber per day.

- *High fiber* indicates that one serving has at least 5 grams of dietary fiber.

- *Good Source of Fiber*. The food product has 2.5 grams to 4.9 grams fiber per serving.

- *More* or *Added Fiber*. The product contains at least 2.5 grams fiber per serving.

- *Sugar*. The grams of sugar in a food can be naturally occurring or added. Check the ingredient list to find out. In good selections, the total grams of carbohydrate in a food serving should be more than twice the amount of sugar grams. If it isn't, leave it on the grocer's shelf.

- *Sugar Free* means there's less than 1/2 gram of sugar per serving.

- *Fat*. This number is determined by adding the grams of saturated fat + grams of polyunsaturated fat + grams of monounsaturated fat.

- *Reduced fat*. The item contains at least 25 percent less total fat than the regular product.

- *Light fat*. The product has 50% less fat than its regular counterpart.

- *Low Fat*. The food contains 3 grams of fat (or less) in a serving.

- *Fat Free*. The food contains 1/2 gram of fat (or less) per serving.

- *With lighter, reduced, low-fat and fat-free products*, pay special attention to other ingredients. When the fat is removed from many recipes, salt and/or sugar are sometimes added back to enhance flavor. This can result in a fat-free or low-fat product that actually has more calories than the regular version.

- *Sat Fat*. Saturated fat is solid at room temperature, e.g. butter, chicken skin, visible fat on a steak, lard, shortening. Less than 10% of your daily calories should be from saturated fats, which are derived mainly from animal products. The saturated fat from animal foods is a primary source of cholesterol. A few plant oils such as coconut and palm are saturated.

- *Sodium*. For most people, the daily recommendation for sodium is 2400 mg. Try to find an average of 240 mg sodium in each of your daily servings.

- *Light in Sodium*. The product has one half of the sodium of its counterparts.

Understanding the Ingredients List

Ingredients are also found on the product label, listed in order of decreasing weight in the food product. If the list begins with sugar (e.g. white sugar, corn syrup, sucrose etc.) or saturated fats and oils, you might want to leave it on the grocer's shelf. Also, a shorter ingredient list often means the product is more natural. A long list of ingredients with a plethora of chemicals and preservatives listed is probably a good product to leave on the store shelf.

Start in the Produce Section

The most important change most people need to make is putting more fruits and vegetables into their shopping carts and their daily diet. The goal is to eat 4 cups fruit/veggies each day, leaning more heavily toward veggies. Tips for shopping for produce:

- *Follow the rainbow*. Different colors of fruits and vegetables mean they contain different phytonutrients, so stock up on all colors.

- *Limit fruit portions to 1/2 cup if you're trying to lose weight.*

- *Bananas are high in starch and calories, so remember that 1/2 medium banana is one serving.* Brush plantains with a little olive oil and grill 'em to enjoy fruit in a savory way.

- *Packaged veggies and fruits may be worth the extra moulah for convenience sake*, if you don't have time to clean them yourself (and it means you'll skip veggies and fruits otherwise).

- *Steer away from veggies with a hard exterior: corn, peas and white potatoes.* They're starchy and contain less water.

- *Sweet potatoes are A-OK.* Sweet potatoes contain almost twice as much fiber as other types of potatoes. They are also high in vitamin B6 and potassium (potassium plays a role in lowering blood pressure and is an important electrolyte), rich in vitamins A, C and E, and a great source of manganese, a trace mineral that helps metabolize carbohydrates. Limit sweet potatoes to 1/2 cup servings, and don't eat them every day.

- *Go green.* Cucumber, broccoli, cabbage, Brussels sprouts, Swiss chard, fennel and kale are all fabulous greens. Blanch kale and rinse in cold water to release the bitterness.

- *Artichokes.* Choose artichokes with petals still tightly closed, they are typically more fresh and tender than artichokes with loose or opened petals. Steam or boil artichokes for 25 to 40 minutes or until the outer leaves can easily be removed.

- *Avocados, the "good" fat.* Good fats add vitamins and help us feel full. They carry flavor and can make our foods taste more robust. One quarter of a medium avocado is 50 calories and a great addition to any salad or sandwich.

- *Grab the herbs.* Herbs are practically no calories, but pack flavor. Any herb that comes in a big bunch (basil, cilantro) is typically not as intense in flavor. Tarragon, thyme and others that are packed in small containers are big on flavor, so you won't need as much of them. To keep basil fresh, wrap the bunch in a paper towel, sprinkle with water, and sit loosely in a plastic bag.

- *Mushrooms, an absolute must-have.* Mushrooms are nearly all water and contain few calories, plus they are loaded with nutrients, flavor and texture.

- *Newbie produce shoppers, you are better off shopping a few times a week in the beginning.* Novice produce eaters tend to overbuy in the beginning, leading to excess waste.

When to Go Organic

Organic foods are foods that have not been treated with pesticides. Typically, organic foods are more expensive than regular foods. Thin-skinned fruits and vegetables, such as berries and leafy greens, more easily absorb pesticides and should be purchased organic if you can afford to do so. If you're on a budget, there are some vegetables that because of their hard-skinned exterior don't necessarily need to be purchased organic.

Each year, the Environmental Working Group (ewg.org), a health research and advocacy organization, puts together a list of foods known to be laden with pesticides that should be either purchased and eaten organically or grown in your own garden. The group estimates that individuals can reduce their exposure to pesticides by 80% when switching to organic foods. The USDA sets allowable pesticide residue limits it deems safe, and produce for sale in your grocery store should meet USDA standards.

According to the Environmental Working Group, you should try to buy and eat *organic* versions of these foods (if you can) as they tend to hang onto pesticide residue[26]:

- *Apples*. Pesticide residue is also found in apple juice and apple sauce. Peeling apples may reduce exposure but you're also peeling away many nutrients.

- *Celery*. If you can't find organic celery, safer alternatives include broccoli, radishes, onions and bok choy.

- *Cherry tomatoes*.

- *Cucumbers*. Skin can be laced with pesticides. Peeling skin can help.

- *Grapes*... and raisins. (For this reason you may want to opt for organic wines as well.)

- *Sweet bell peppers and hot peppers*.

- *Peaches.*
- *Strawberries.* Frozen strawberries have less residue, but opt for packages with no added sugar. Kiwi and pineapples are good alternatives.
- *Spinach.*
- *Kale.* Organic kale is readily available (which can mean reasonable prices). Alternatives include cabbage, asparagus and broccoli.
- *Collard Greens.* If you can't find organic greens, Brussels sprouts, dandelion greens and cabbage are good alternatives.
- *Zucchini.*
- *Lettuce.*
- *Blueberries.*

If the cost of organic isn't within your budget, these foods are typically low in pesticides:

- *Onions*
- *Pineapple*
- *Avocado*
- *Asparagus*
- *Mango*
- *Papayas*
- *Eggplant*
- *Cantaloupe*
- *Watermelon*
- *Sweet Potatoes*
- *Grapefruit*
- *Mushrooms*

Just Say No... To Juice

People ask me all the time about juicing. I don't recommend drinking juices - they have very little fiber and typically a higher concentration of sugars than the actual fruit (1 cup of juice may equal several pieces of fruit sugar-wise). *Drinking fruit* makes your blood sugar go up, come down, and then you're hungry again. *Eating fruit* is more satisfying (the crunching and chewing makes you feel like you've eaten something substantial, and whole fruits take longer to digest than juices), provides your body with fiber (which keeps you feeling full longer), and (ounce for ounce) contains about half of the calories of juice. When eating a piece of fruit, pair it with a protein (mozzarella stick, Greek yogurt, a slice of turkey) to keep your blood sugar from rising quickly and to help it come down more slowly. Plus, protein makes you feel fuller.

Meats, Poultry and Fish

The right cuts of meats and poultry provide tons of protein while limiting fat. And in addition to being a good source of protein, fish provides omega-3s, fatty acids that are essential to a multitude of body and brain functions. Tips for selecting the best meat, fish and poultry options:

- *Chicken - white meat's the right meat*. Dark meat has intra-muscular fat; white meat is the leanest part of the bird. If you can afford organic, all the better. Make sure your chicken is skinless, and if buying a packaged brand, carefully read the label to check for added salt water. If salt is added, leave it on the store shelf.

- *The other white meat - pork*. Pork tenderloin is as lean as a chicken breast! Stay away from marinated offerings to avoid added salt and sugars.

- *Go lean on beef*. Top round, filet mignon and flank steak are the leanest cuts. Trim away any visible fat. Make sure ground beef is at least 95% lean.

- *Try bison*. It's absolutely delicious with a very mild gamey taste. And because it's usually grass-fed, it will be higher in omega-3s, too.

- *Opt for wild fish rather than farmed*. No matter how well-tended the farm, most farmed fish are swimming in water that's generally not as clean as open water. (The exception is fish farmed in the clear, frigid waters of Norway.)

- *Shellfish is OK - choose wild.*

- *Frozen fish is a fantastic, on-hand option*. Thaw it, then pat it dry before cooking to keep it from getting watery.

- *So is canned salmon*, which is usually always wild.

Dairy Options

Dairy products provide us with a multitude of protein options. So unless you're lactose intolerant, incorporate dairy into your daily regimen (there are lactose-free milk options for those with lactose issues). If you're approaching menopause (or already there), you need to increase your dairy intake to keep calcium and protein levels up. Tips for buying dairy:

- *Go organic with milk and eggs*. Highly recommended, especially if you have kids.

- *Buy the carton with the screw top*. The screw top guarantees a longer shelf life.

- *Use 1% milk instead of cream in your coffee (unless you prefer it black)*. 1% milk has more body than nonfat to help make coffee taste creamier.

- *Go Greek*. Greek yogurt contains twice the protein as regular yogurt and half the carb.

- *Fat-free cottage cheese is a great mixer*. A half cup of cottage cheese mixed with 1/2 cup salsa (or fruit, veggies, etc.) makes a great snack.

- *Opt for fat-free ricotta.*

- *String cheese or cheese sticks are an ideal snack.* Quick, easy and portable.

- *Don't forget goats!* There are plenty of scrumptious goat dairy products on the market today, including cheese, yogurt and kefir, which are loaded with calcium and protein.

Canned and Packaged Goods

Opt for these smart choices:

- *Fire-roasted tomatoes.* They add flavor! Try them in BBQ sauce, chili and pasta sauces.

- *Water-packed tuna and salmon.* My favorites are Sustainable Seas and Wild Planet, sustainably harvested wild fish.

- *Corn and whole-wheat tortillas.* Look at the label to make sure that "whole wheat" or "whole grain" is the first ingredient. If "white or wheat flour" is the first ingredient, they aren't truly whole wheat. You can freeze tortillas and thaw as needed. Need to watch for fat, though.

- *Whole-grain pasta.*

- *Cereals with at least 5 grams fiber per serving and under 5 grams of sugar.*

- *Steel-cut or old-fashioned oatmeal.* (gluten-free options are available)

- *Whole-grain bread.* Look at fiber counts on the label and get the bread highest in fiber. Ezekiel Bread (in the freezer case) is a good option. Freeze bread so that you use only as needed.

- *Pre-cooked and pre-packaged single-serve rice.* Packaged in a single serving so that you don't eat too much. Opt for brown rice.

Fine-tuning Serving Size

Consuming appropriate portion sizes is essential to a healthful, balanced diet. But our eyes often deceive us (hence, the well-used adage "*my eyes were bigger than my stomach*"), especially when we're hungry! Something as simple as the amount of meat or cheese layered on a sandwich can easily add up to extra fat calories we don't even realize we're eating.

In order to gauge the calorie content of meals and snacks, you'll need to pay very close attention to serving size. That's why it's important to measure and weigh your food, so you know **EXACTLY** how many calories you're eating and drinking.

Essential tools for accurately measuring foods:

- *Liquid measuring cup* (2-cup capacity)
- *Set of dry measuring cups* (1-cup, 1/2 cup, 1/3 cup, and 1/4 cup sizes)
- *Set of measuring spoons* (1 tablespoon, 1 teaspoon, 1/2 teaspoon, 1/4 teaspoon)
- *Food scale* (measuring in pounds, ounces and grams – most ingredient measurements are in ounces, but foods concentrated in calories are often measured in grams). See Shopping Resources on page 148.
- *Calculator* (for tallying calories). You probably have one on your phone.

Tips for measuring foods:

- *Weigh and measure food <u>after</u> cooking*. The weight of food typically changes when cooked. Food that contains water or liquids weigh less after cooking, while dry cereals and grains can double or triple in both weight and volume after being cooked in liquid.

- *Read nutrition labels on packaged foods.* They will guide you on portion sizes.

- *Pay attention to "serving size."* Labeled serving size can be much smaller than what *you* consider a serving size.

- *Calculate calorie counts of favorite meals and note in your journal.* For meals you make and eat frequently (most of us eat the same breakfast several days a week) you'll only need to measure and weigh once, calculate the calories, and record the calorie count

Conversion Table for Measuring Portion Sizes

Teaspoon	Tablespoon	Cups	Pints/quarts gallons	Fluid ounce	Milliliter
1/4 teaspoon					1 ml
1/2 teaspoon					2 ml
1 teaspoon	1/3 tablespoon				5 ml
3 teaspoons	1 tablespoon	1/16 cup		1/2 oz.	15 ml
6 teaspoons	2 tablespoons	1/8 cup		1 oz.	30 ml
12 teaspoons	4 tablespoons	1/4 cup		2 oz.	60 ml
16 teaspoons	5 1/3 tablespoons	1/3 cup		2 1/2 oz.	75 ml
24 teaspoons	8 tablespoons	1/2 cup		4 oz.	125 ml
32 teaspoons	10 2/3 tablespoons	2/3 cup		5 oz.	150 ml
36 teaspoons	12 tablespoons	3/4 cup		6 oz.	175 ml
48 teaspoons	16 tablespoons	1 cup	1/2 pint	8 oz.	237 ml
		2 cups	1 pint	16 oz.	473 ml
		3 cups		24 oz.	710 ml
		4 cups	1 quart	32 oz.	946 ml
		8 cups	1/2 gallon	64 oz.	1893 ml
		16 cups	1 gallon	128 oz.	3785 ml

in your journal. The next time you have that same breakfast - voilà! - no need to measure or calculate, you'll already have the calorie count on hand to record into your journal.

Cookware that Puts Flavor (not Calories) First

Nonstick cookware is perfect for calorie-counting cooks. Try to prepare or warm up foods with minimal added fats. Basic cookware to keep on hand:

- *Ovenproof skillet or sauté pan* (with a lid)
- *7-quart (or bigger) stock or soup pot* (with a lid)
- *Saucepans* (1-quart and 3-quart, with lids)
- *Several 15x10-inch baking sheets*
- *Roasting pan* (with bottom rack)
- *9x13-inch casserole or baking dish*
- *Steamer* (Some pots and pans come with a steamer insert, or you can buy a freestanding steamer basket that fits the pot you are using.)
- *Colander*
- *Nonstick muffin pans* (regular and miniature sizes)

Essential Kitchen Tools

In addition to the many traditional tools needed in the kitchen, some not-so-traditional essentials are a tremendous help in keeping calorie counts down. Items to consider for your *Losing Big* kitchen:

- *Slotted spoon.* Helpful for lifting items out of their cooking liquids.
- *Squeeze bottles.* Aim, shoot and squeeze small amounts of sauces, doling out just the right portion size.
- *Spray bottle.* Spritz a minimal amount of oil into a pan.

- *Handheld zester and grater*. More than 50% of vitamin C in citrus fruits is in the peel, so add a dash of zest to your tea, salad or hot cereal. Finely grated hard cheeses add a dusting of flavor without overdoing fat and calories.

- *Blender*. For producing healthful, low-calorie smoothies and smooth, silky soups.

- *Baking liners*. Avoid buttering or adding extra oil to baking sheets by using parchment paper or reusable nonstick baking mats made of flexible silicone-based material. Parchment paper is also great for wrapping foods before oven baking to lock in moisture and flavor.

- *Egg pricker*. This little gadget pricks a tiny hole in an egg's shell. Air (but no egg!) escapes, keeping the egg from cracking while it cooks and making a hardboiled egg much easier to peel.

Cooking with Less Fat

When you cook food, heat can be applied in primarily two ways: dry heat or wet heat. Dry heat surrounds your ingredients - whether in the oven or on a grill - with hot, dry air. Wet-heat methods use hot liquid to cook food. Each of the following dry and wet heat techniques don't rely on oodles of oil or fats, so they will add flavor - but not many calories - to your dishes.

Dry-heat cooking tips:

- *Baking*. Perfectly baked food retains moisture and optimal flavor development. Oven baking requires a steady temperature, usually between 200 and 400 degrees.

- *Broiling*. Food needs to be placed directly beneath a heat source - in your oven, that's either an open flame or the top heating element - usually at temps above 450 degrees.

- *Grilling*. A quick cooking method using high temperatures over an open heat source. Can be stovetop or outdoor grill. Be sure to cut away any portion of food that becomes blackened to avoid ingesting dangerous carcinogens.

- *Roasting*. Cook foods in an open pan. Don't crowd the pan; allow hot air to circulate evenly.

- *Toasting*. Quickly heat and brown food surfaces by placing food near a heat source. Great for spices, grains, nuts and seeds.

Wet-heat cooking methods and tips:

- *Blanching*. Veggies or fruits are blanched to soften, partially cook or fully cook, or to remove a strong taste. Food is dipped into boiling water, removed after a timed interval, and then placed into iced water or under cold running water to stop the cooking process.

- *Boiling*. If you use vegetable stock rather than water as the base liquid, you'll instantly boost flavor.

- *Poaching*. Cook food in a small amount of boiling liquid, usually just enough to cover the food. Again, using broth instead of water will kick the flavor up a notch.

- *Pressure cooking*. Cooks food more quickly, drastically reducing meal preparation time. The specialized heavy pot with sealed lid allows pressure to build up in the pot when it's placed over heat.

- *Steaming*. Instead of using plain water to steam food, create flavor - without calories - by adding herbs, spices or tea leaves to the pot.

- *Stewing*. Cover food with a bare minimum of liquid and cook it gently for a long period of time in a covered pot. Flavors in the ingredients will blend, infusing the liquid with richness.

Somewhere in between dry- and wet-cooking methods:

- *Braising*. Brown ingredients by roasting, baking or grilling, then cook in a covered pot with a small amount of liquid to retain moisture.

- *Sautéing*. Derived from the French verb *sauter*, meaning "to jump," sautéing involves cooking ingredients in a shallow pan over high heat and shaking the pan intermittently to make the food "jump." To minimize the use of fat, opt for a nonstick pan and - if you must - coat with a mist (from your spray bottle) of oil.

- *Microwaving*. Electromagnetic radiation cooks foods swiftly without requiring fat, but ingredients often lose moisture, change texture and don't brown. I use my microwave to heat milk for my coffee or warm up frozen foods and leftovers

Chapter Ten
SOS! I've Done Everything Right, But...

Feeling Stuck?

You've been eating healthful meals, monitoring your daily calorie intake, getting plenty of exercise and are experiencing great results... but suddenly... you're stuck! You've either hit a plateau or overindulged (it happens!) and need to get back on track.

Help is here! The SOS Plan is a streamlined, *temporary* solution that delivers essential nutrition and a noticeable drop in weight. Core concepts of the SOS Plan:

- *Maintain your overall calorie budget*
- *Increase lean protein intake* - from fish, poultry and meat - to 35% of calories
- *Reduce carbohydrate intake* to 40% of calories, and limit these carbs to fresh fruits and vegetables *only*
- *Eliminate whole grains* (remember, this is only temporary)
- *Reduce or eliminate legumes*
- *Maintain your intake of healthy fats* at 25% of total calories. The menus beginning on page 97 in *Appendix 2* will illustrate the right balance of carbs, protein and good fat for each meal and snack.
- *Limit the time period and frequency of the SOS plan* to no more than four weeks at a time, and no more than three times a year

Why is this combination so effective for weight loss? The key lies in the *type* of calories consumed - a shift toward protein and reduction in carbohydrates. And there's a psychological component, too; by shaking up your eating routine, you're likely to refocus and recharge on your habits and identify areas of slippage.

Protein: The Key to Rapid Weight Loss

Protein intake can affect weight loss dramatically for a couple of reasons:

- *Protein burns more calories*. Our bodies actually burn calories to extract nutrients from the foods we eat, a process called the "thermic effect." More calories are burned processing proteins than either fats or carbohydrates. Even upping your lean protein intake just 5%, as the SOS Plan recommends, can cause a shift in your diet's overall thermic effect - burning more calories overall.

- *Protein makes you feel full longer*. High-protein foods produce a sensation of fullness, or satiety. Researchers are still discovering why protein uniquely produces this effect, but the weight-loss results are convincing. It may be due to the fact that protein is metabolized more slowly, causing blood sugar levels to remain stable longer, affecting neurotransmitters in the brain that promote satiety.

Come Clean with Your Carbs

While the SOS Plan increases protein intake, it decreases carbohydrate consumption, by (temporarily) eliminating grains and cereals. Carbohydrates continue to play the leading role, but there's one key difference - *all your carbohydrate calories should come from fruits and vegetables*. It's all about balance. Diets too high in protein and extremely low in carbs can strain the kidneys. There are several reasons for focusing on fruits and vegetables:

- *Fruits and veggies provide the highest nutrient bang for calorie buck*. Nonstarchy fruits and vegetables are low in calories but loaded with the fiber and antioxidant vitamins that promote health.

- *Produce is filling*. Many varieties of fresh produce are high in water content and fiber, meaning you can eat plenty for just a few calories - helping you fill up and feel satisfied. A cup of brown rice has 216 calories, while the same amount of chopped cabbage has just 21 calories, giving you plenty of crunchy filling for minimal calorie investment.

The Result: A Notable Drop

The combined effect of increased protein intake and reduced carbohydrate consumption can have a powerful, temporary effect on the scale. Why? Well, for each gram of carbohydrate the cells in your body store, they store 4 grams of water. Initial weight loss when eliminating carbohydrates from your diet is mostly water weight (less carbohydrates, less water as well). When you decrease the amount of carbohydrates you eat, your body burns glycogen, a quick energy supply stored in your muscles and liver alongside a supply of water. When you burn the glycogen, the water is excreted.

To see long-term success with weight loss, it's important to consume fewer total calories, but to include all food groups to maximize nutritional value.

Extra Boost: Intensify Your Exercise Routine

The SOS Plan is a perfect opportunity to kick things up a notch and shake up your exercise routine, too. Try some high-intensity exercise (*see Chapter Seven, Build and Burn–Exercise for Weight Loss*) like interval training or increase your frequency of resistance training by 1 or 2 times per week.

Remember, the SOS Plan is a *temporary* solution to weight-loss plateaus and occasional over-indulgences, **NOT** a long-term plan! Seeing the numbers move in the right direction on the scale may just provide the rewarding feeling that can jump-start your commitment to weight loss.

Chapter Eleven
Eating and Exercising Away From Home

Life is Like a Box of (Low Calorie and Low Fat) Chocolates

Congratulations! You're eating calorie-appropriate meals and snacks several times a day, using a food journal, and regularly exercising with resistance and intensity. You've successfully balanced *Losing Big* food and exercise like clockwork and you're seeing results.

But, as we all know, life happens. And, like that box of chocolates, you never know what you're going to get! An unexpected long workday, a last-minute business trip, a holiday party or even a vacation can derail your routine and healthful habits. The trick to navigating unforeseen glitches – like having to work late – is to always have a "plan B" in place to help you adapt to whatever chaos life throws your way.

At the Office

The office is a potential minefield when it comes to healthful eating. Long hours, business lunches, doughnuts in the break room, birthday cakes, vending machines and latte runs are just a few of the booby traps you'll need to side step on a weekly basis. When navigating workplace eating, being prepared is half the battle.

Tips to staying on track at work:

- *Pack snacks*. A bowl of fruit at your desk and pre-measured individual servings of nuts in your desk drawer are good to keep on hand. Most 100 calorie pre-packaged snack packs are simply smaller servings of junk food – avoid them! Quality calories are key.

- *Nuts!*

  ❖ Pistachios contain a plant chemical called anthocyanin, which is thought to boost the immune system. They are lower in fat than most other types of tree nuts. Pistachios have 160 calories in a one ounce serving which equals 49 nuts.

❖ Walnuts are high in omega-3 fatty acids, which are thought to help slow the aging process, encourage healthy cholesterol levels, possibly reduce the need for steroids in conditions such as rheumatoid arthritis or inflammatory bowel disease, and possibly delay or prevent the onset of Alzheimer's... among a host of other benefits.

❖ Almonds contain more calcium than other nuts; a 1-ounce serving delivers 7% of the daily value for calcium based on a 2,000-calorie diet.

❖ Raw or dry-roasted cashews or pecans are high in immune-boosting zinc. Go nuts!

• *Fridge snacks*, too. If there's kitchen and cupboard space, create a small stockpile of healthful options such as peanut butter, mozzarella sticks or yogurt. Low-calorie, high-protein/carb snacks can help combat stress: An apple with peanut butter, fat-free Greek yogurt with fresh fruit and an orange with a slice of turkey are just a few options.

• *Watch the caffeine.* Remember that caffeine's a stimulant, and when it wears off you can feel foggy or groggy and less able to deal with your daily grind. Instead reach for water or a cup of herbal tea. *And don't forget - four cups of green tea a day can kick up your metabolism by 80 calories.*[27] *- it all adds up!*

• *Hydrate with water.* Water transports oxygen and nutrients to tissues and can help you feel refreshed. Keep a pitcher or large drinking container at your desk. Better still, replenish from the water cooler frequently; the walk and stretch will do you good.

• *Breathe - don't eat - on your break.* A quick walk around the block or simply standing and stretching between tasks will help relieve tension and keep you away from the candy bowl.

- *Plan for business lunches*. Research the menu when you prepare for the meeting, or have a go-to item in mind for lunches out - like broiled fish or a green salad with skinless chicken.

- *Refresh your commute*. Change it up to de-stress or include exercise. Take the ferry or bus and relax - read the newspaper, listen to music, meditate or plan your day. Walk, run or bike to and from work, rather than drive. If you drive daily, park several blocks away or at the far end of the lot and walk.

- *Stand when you can*. Stand up to take phone calls or raise your computer so you're standing, rather than sitting, when doing computer work.

- *Stash workout clothes at your desk and be familiar with local exercise options*. Business lunch cancels unexpectedly? Use the time to take a run, attend a noon-time yoga class, or work out at a local gym.

- *Take the stairs*. Anytime you can. Enough said.

Eating Out

My top tip for successful weight loss is to **LOSE THE WHITE STUFF**. The easiest way to make this change at home is to avoid putting white stuff - including white rice, white flour, white pasta and white sugar - in your grocery cart. Eating healthfully when dining out, however, is challenging but not impossible. If your family has a favorite go-to restaurant, request whole grains and healthy options. Restaurants want to please their customers, especially regulars.

Tips for ordering on (and off!) the menu:

- *Be assertive*. When exploring the menu, ask your server how items are prepared (fried? steamed? sautéed?).

- *Have it your way!* It's **OK** to request that your chicken, fish and/or vegetables be prepared without added oil or buttery sauces; ask to have them baked, broiled or grilled instead.

- *Choose takeout wisely.* Steer clear of fast-food drive-thrus. Opt for stir-fry, sashimi or sushi with brown rice and order steamed brown rice and plenty of veggies.

- *Go whole grain... with everything possible.* Ask for whole-grain rolls, crackers, tortillas (corn or whole wheat – instead of white flour). Request whole-grain pasta or whole-grain pizza crust.

- *Choose oatmeal or whole-grain bagels* instead of white bread or white bagels for breakfast.

- *Ask for brown rice* instead of white rice when ordering Chinese/Indian food or sushi.

- *You may balk at the thought of asking your local restaurant for whole-grain bread or brown rice sushi.* But if no one ever requests it, nothing will change and white stuff will continue to be the standard.

- *Whole grains on the side.* Choose whole grains for your starch sides – polenta, brown rice, wild rice, bulgur or tabbouleh – instead of potatoes or white rice. And remember 1/2 cup is a serving. If you have trouble with your willpower (who doesn't?) ask them to bring only 1/2 cup with your order.

- *Ask wait staff to check the ounce size on bar pours.* There can be a big difference between a standard 5-ounce wine pour and a "regular customer" oversized pour.

Have Healthy Snacks, Will Travel

Vacations can be good for the soul by reducing stress, promoting balance and providing rejuvenation. And work travel... well... it's just plain necessary sometimes. But even the best-laid travel plans need tweaking to keep you on your health and fitness track.

Tips for staying healthy on the road:

- *Comfortable shoes a must.* Take stairs or walk through the airport (rather than using people movers).

- *Find a hotel with a fitness center or pool.* Or talk with the concierge about walking or running routes, or the location (and safety) of stairs and whether they are appropriate for walking (check on access from floors to make sure doors are unlocked).

- *Better yet, choose a wellness-friendly hotel; they make it easier to stay healthy while on the road.* Wellness-friendly hotels are growing increasingly popular. I recently began working with Omni Hotels & Resorts because of their incredible Healthy Travel program, ranging from gym equipment in guest rooms to healthier items on kids and room service menus.

- *Plan for plane time.* Pack TSA-friendly snack food: nuts, cut veggies and fresh fruit (note that yogurt, while well-intentioned, isn't TSA friendly, but you can pick it up gate-side). If your flight spans meal time, pick up a healthy meal - salad or turkey sandwich on whole wheat - and water inside security and carry it aboard. While in flight, hydrate, hydrate and then hydrate again with bottled water, at least one cup for every hour in the air.

- *Pack snacks for the car.* Healthful snacks can be difficult to find on the road. If you have the room, carry a cooler, fill it with double-bagged ice to keep food cold but dry, and then carry fruits, veggies, sandwich fixings and water.

- *Skip the junk food.* Save calorie splurges for unique local fare.

- *Step away from the minibar.* Nothing good - diet-wise - can come from raiding the minibar! If you must... read labels!

- *Avoid the buffet.* Opt for traditional restaurants rather than tempting all-you-can-eat diet disasters zones. If buffet is your only option, choose a small plate.

- *Eat family style.* At a restaurant, order healthful dishes and one single splurge specialty - such as a local favorite or dessert - and pass the plates so everyone can have a small taste.

- *Get a room with a kitchenette.* Then hit the grocery store on arrival. Brew your own coffee, have a healthful breakfast and pack a lunch to go to save on calories (and restaurant bills!).

- *Park it...* the car, that is. Walk around town instead. You can easily log a couple of miles each day exploring.

- *Build activity into every day.* Vegging out is part of the deal, but try to dedicate a few hours a day to physical activity, whether a walking tour, snorkeling or a night of dancing.

Special Events and Parties

From weddings to family reunions to holiday get-togethers, parties can be a healthful-eating challenge! In the whirl of chatter, good company and alcohol, you can easily lose track of how much you've tasted and nibbled.

Tips for beating the buffet:

- *Eat first.* Never go to a party hungry. Eat half a sandwich or yogurt with fruit before you go.

- *Sip smart.* Avoid alcohol if possible. Alcohol can hinder willpower and makes it much easier to eat too much or not make the right choices. Drink ice water or a spritzer with club soda and lime. If you must imbibe, drink wine or champagne. A 4-ounce glass of wine has approximately 100 calories.

- *Stand up.* Don't pile on a plateful and hunker down in a corner for a feeding frenzy. Standing burns more calories than sitting.

- *Work the room.* When you're tempted to have seconds, engage in conversation instead.

- *Focus on finger foods.* Bite-sized treats may be rich, but the small size limits the calorie impact.

- *Work out beforehand.* When you put a party on your calendar, schedule exercise the same day to offset the extra calories.

Whetting Your Whistle, Holiday- and Party-Style

It can be difficult to avoid consuming cocktails and wine during the holiday season. But most alcoholic beverages are full of calories and not much else of nutritional value. And a few drinks can break the bank on your calorie budget. Traditional eggnog, for instance, has 343 calories and 19 grams of fat (11 grams saturated fat) per cup! So how to stick to a healthful diet during the holidays and still enjoy a libation (or two)?

Tips for holiday and party drinking:

- *Do drink conservatively.* Limit yourself to one or two drinks interspersed with water and healthful nibbles.

- *Don't quench your thirst with a martini. Do drink a big glass or two of water prior to drinking alcohol.* Water makes you feel full and provides your body with the hydration it needs for optimal body function.

- *Do choose wine.* Wine has calories, but no fat, and contains antioxidants (especially when it's red wine!). A 4.1-ounce glass of champagne has 78 calories, while a 5-ounce glass of red wine has 127 calories and the antioxidant resveratrol. Just make sure you're drinking a single serving.

- *Do try a wine spritzer.* Wine mixed with sparkling water is a festive drinking option, with half the calories.

- *Do opt for faux cocktails.* If you're self-conscious about navigating a party without a cocktail (or just want to avoid people trying to pour you drinks all night) try sparkling water with a slice of lemon or lime. No one will know it's not a gin and tonic!

- *Do offset indulgences with exercise.* Before burning protein, carbs or fat calories, your body will burn off alcohol. That means that if you choose to drink, you need to spend extra time working out.

- *Skip the cream.* Drinks like eggnog or Irish cream liqueurs are loaded with fat and calories.

Appendix 1
Shopping List

Cheryl's Shopping Tips

Buy less, waste less

Shop more often instead of stocking up and allowing some items to go to waste.

Ask for it!

If your store doesn't carry everything you need (such as fat-free Greek-style yogurt, fat-free ricotta cheese, and low-sodium sliced turkey breast), ask your grocer to order it.

Shop with a list and stick to it!

A list curbs impulsive purchases and cuts down grocery bills.

What to Buy?

When initially stocking your kitchen the *Losing Big* way, purchase the shelf-stable items on these lists to have on hand. Then a few times a week, purchase perishables needed to complete a day or three's worth of recipes. When purchasing perishables follow the guidelines and suggestions provided in *Chapter Eight, Stocking Your Kitchen, on page 61.*

Keep it simple

Avoid foods that contain more than five ingredients, artificial ingredients or ingredients you can't pronounce.

Herbs and Spices
Fresh

Nothing beats the flavor of tomatoes topped with freshly chopped basil or the herbaceous kick of parsley added to whole grains. I recommend buying the following herbs fresh whenever possible. Unless you grow them yourself, you may want to buy fresh herbs when needed, as they don't last long.

- √ Basil
- √ Cilantro
- √ Chives
- √ Dill
- √ Garlic
- √ Ginger
- √ Italian flat-leaf parsley
- √ Mint
- √ Oregano
- √ Tarragon
- √ Thyme

Fresh Herb Storage

Even perishable fresh herbs can last two weeks or longer when stored properly. Follow these steps to preserve fresh herbs as long as possible:

1. Gently wash the herbs immediately and then drain or spin them, using a salad spinner.
2. Separate the stalks, removing any wilted/rotten leaves, and then snip off the bottom of the stems.
3. Either place the clipped ends of the herbs in a jar of water in the fridge (like a flower bouquet in a vase) or wrap herbs in a just-damp paper towel and seal them in a plastic bag. You can also find products on the market called herb keepers that take the guesswork out of storing herbs and that can help you keep fresh herbs on hand conveniently.

Dried

When fresh herbs from the list in the preceding section aren't readily available, be sure you have their dried counterparts in the cupboard. Buy dried herbs and spices in small quantities, as they tend to lose their potency in about one year's time. Dried herbs are more concentrated than fresh, so use them sparingly in recipes. Let taste guide you, but a good ratio is one teaspoon of dried herbs is equivalent to a tablespoon of fresh.

Ratio of Dried vs. Fresh Herbs
1 teaspoon dried = 1 tablespoon fresh

In addition to those listed previously, I also recommend investing in the following dried herbs.

- √ Bay leaves
- √ Marjoram
- √ Rosemary
- √ Sage

Spices

Even small amounts of herbs and spices deliver a powerful punch of flavor and can zip up any dish. I keep my spice rack stocked with the following flavorful spices.

- √ Allspice
- √ Anise
- √ Black pepper
- √ Cardamom
- √ Celery seed
- √ Chili powder
- √ Cinnamon
- √ Cloves
- √ Crushed red pepper flakes
- √ Coriander
- √ Cumin
- √ Curry powder
- √ Fennel seed
- √ Ground ginger

- ✓ Mustard seed
- ✓ Ground mustard
- ✓ Paprika (hot and sweet, smoked and unsmoked)
- ✓ Poppy seed
- ✓ Spice blends (low-sodium or sodium-free options)
- ✓ Turmeric

Drill for Oil

Knowing how to use healthful oils in your cooking can actually make your food taste more robust. Different varieties of oil can impart very different flavors, and their fat content adds richness to a dish and promotes a feeling of satiety, or fullness, when you eat it that can turn a quick bowl of grains into a satisfying supper.

Good Fat

Choose good fats such as polyunsaturated and monounsaturated fats found in foods like nuts, seeds, olive oils and avocados.

There are two main categories of healthful oils: vegetable oils (including seed oils) and nut oils.

When cooking, it's up to you what oil you want to use. Different oils have different smoke points, and you don't want oil to smoke in the pan. The smoke point for grapeseed oil, for example, is about 420 degrees, while flaxseed oil is only 220 degrees (meaning you don't want to cook with flaxseed oil).

Use grapeseed or olive oil as your everyday cooking oil and then add a dash of the more exotic and pricey oils for added flavor.

Vegetable Oils

These oils are extracted from plant matter. My favorite is olive oil, a staple of the Mediterranean diet that has been used since 3000 BCE. Olive oil has a slightly grassy, vegetal flavor.

√ Olive Oil: "Extra-virgin" and "virgin" oils come from the first pressings and are unrefined; their flavors are purest for salad dressings and other uncooked sauces. Lower grades (such as "semi-fine" or "pure") are less flavorful, but withstand high temperatures better. Olive oil not only contains HDL-boosting compounds, but also vitamin E and antioxidants.

Seed Oils

A subset of vegetable oils, seed oils are made from pressed plant seeds and deliver highly concentrated nutrients and flavors in small doses.

√ Flaxseed oil (low smoke point): Contains heart-healthy omega-3 fatty acids, this oil is mild enough to be used in salad dressings, although its low smoke point makes it undesirable for cooking.

√ Grapeseed oil: This slightly nutty oil contains antioxidant properties and withstands heat well. It can be infused with herbs to create an aromatic blend. Grapeseed oil has one of the lowest levels of saturated fats of all oils.

√ Sesame oil (high smoke point): Both the light and dark varieties of this oil are extracted from sesame seeds; the darker variety lends a pronounced, nutty flavor to dishes. A common ingredient in Asian cooking, sesame oil has a high smoke point, which makes it a popular option for stir-frying. Sesame oil is high in polyunsaturated fats.

Nut Oils

Like the nuts from which they're produced, nut oils are a good source of beneficial fats. Nut oils tend to be pricier than vegetable oils, so they come in smaller bottles. Investing in a few good-quality nut oils is worth it, because they add flavor and healthy fats to your dishes. Two of the nut oils I often use are:

- ✓ Walnut oil: This oil has a delicate flavor and is high in omega-3 fatty acids, which promote heart and brain health. It's ideal for salads but doesn't hold up well in high heat.

- ✓ Almond oil: This aromatic oil has a higher smoke point than walnut oil, making it more versatile for use in cooking.

Vinegars and Other Liquid Flavors

Fermentation is the chemical process used to create some of our favorite grown-up beverages, from crisp white wines to hearty ales. But fermentation is also an ally when it comes to flavor: it's the method by which a number of tart, zingy condiments are created. You may think of vinegar as the yang to oil's yin in salad dressings. But this pantry staple – whose name comes from the French term vinaigre, or "sour wine" – can lend its tart, astringent flavor to an array of dishes, from soups to desserts.

Experiment with the following vinegars to add more robust flavor to your dishes and very few calories:

- ✓ Balsamic vinegar: Made from Italian white wine grapes, this luscious purple vinegar is often sweet enough to enjoy on salads without adding oil. Reducing it to a syrup is a quick and easy way to create a sauce that is delicious with fruit.

- ✓ Rice vinegar: A staple in Asian cooking, this extremely mild vinegar adds sweet notes to salad dressings. It is available in seasoned and unseasoned varieties; I recommend using the unseasoned vinegar.

- ✓ Apple cider vinegar: You can use this sweet, fruity vinegar to impart flavor to meat marinades and salads.

Sauces and condiments

Fermented sauces and condiments contribute rich umami (a savory taste) and open a new door to flavor. Because they make foods taste rich without added fat, these condiments are especially useful:

- ✓ Soy sauce: This nutty liquid is made from fermented soybeans and barley or wheat, and is a key flavoring for Asian dishes. Most soy sauces are not gluten-free.

- √ Tamari: Like soy sauce, tamari is made from soybeans, but it has a milder flavor and slightly thicker texture. Check the label: True tamari is fermented without wheat – making it a gluten-free alternative to soy sauce – but because the term "tamari" is sometimes used to describe and market various types of soy sauce, be sure to read the label if you have a gluten allergy.

- √ Fish sauce: Made from the liquid collected from fermented fish. The sauce has the tang of seaweed and a strong fishy taste. It's very popular in Asian cooking.

- √ Worcestershire sauce: Originally a variant of fish sauce, Worcestershire is made from a vinegar base. Current versions of this tangy sauce can still contain anchovies, along with soy sauce, garlic and other spices. Worcestershire sauce is used to flavor meats, gravies, and soups – not to mention Bloody Mary cocktails. Be sure to look for the gluten-free label if that is a concern.

Many of these sauces tend to contain a lot of salt. Choose low-sodium versions when available.

Spreads and Other Items

Always look for lower-salt options for these zesty additions to your pantry. And if you buy condiments rather than make them, choose no-sugar-added varieties.

- √ Capers
- √ Barbecue sauce and ketchup
- √ Fresh salsa
- √ Fruit spreads
- √ Guacamole (fresh, no sour cream added)

- √ Horseradish
- √ Dijon and brown mustards
- √ Pico de gallo
- √ Tabasco sauce
- √ Unsulfured molasses

Appendix 2
The *Losing Big* Plan
Two Weeks Sample Menus

OK, I've shared most of my secrets with you. Let's put them into action. What does a 1,200-calorie (or 1,500- or 1,800-calorie) meal look like? And, more importantly, what does it feel like? The *Losing Big* menu plans are based on an average of 1,200 calories per day. If your calorie needs are a little higher (or lower), you can adjust accordingly.

Adding a glass of 1 percent milk, 6 ounces of fat-free yogurt, one pear or a large apple, or a 4-ounce glass of red wine with dinner will each provide an additional 100 calories.

The two snacks can be scheduled between meals or one *between* meals and one after dinner. For some of you this may be entirely new territory. But really pay attention (and take pictures) of your meals and how you feel afterward.

Your body may need a little time to adjust, but in a couple of weeks, you'll have the hang of this.

For more recipes and menu suggestions, please visit my website at cherylforberg.com

WEEK ONE

DAY 1
1,190 calories

BREAKFAST
1 serving **Cherry Vanilla Granola** (page 118)
1 cup fat-free Greek yogurt
1 cup fat-free milk
8 ounces green tea or water
Black coffee or tea

MID-MORNING SNACK
2 tablespoons hummus
1/2 cup each celery and carrot sticks
8 ounces water or iced green tea with lemon

LUNCH
3 cups shredded romaine lettuce
1/2 cup sliced cucumber
1/2 cup halved cherry tomatoes
3 ounces grilled or roast chicken breast (skinless)
2 tablespoons light **Caesar** dressing
8 ounces water or fat-free milk

MID-AFTERNOON SNACK
1/2 cup plain fat-free Greek-style yogurt topped with 2 tablespoons dried cranberries and 2 tablespoons chopped pecans
1/4 cup blueberries
8 ounces green tea or water

DINNER
4 ounces poached or grilled salmon
6 poached or grilled asparagus spears
1/2 cup quinoa or whole-wheat couscous
Tea or decaf or water

DAY 2
1,250 calories

BREAKFAST
1 cup rolled oats, cooked
1/2 cup fat-free milk or soy milk, 1/2 medium banana, sliced
2 slices (1 ounce) nitrate-free turkey bacon
1 large egg, hard- or soft-boiled
8 ounces water or green tea with a slice of fresh ginger

MID-MORNING SNACK
1/2 cup fat-free ricotta cheese with 1/2 teaspoon vanilla,
1/4 cup blackberries and 2 tablespoons chopped pistachios
Green tea or water

LUNCH
2 servings **Miso Soup with Spinach and Mushrooms** (page 132)
2 cups dark green, leafy salad with 1 tablespoon light balsamic dressing
1 (2-inch) wedge cantaloupe
Iced green tea or water

MID-AFTERNOON SNACK

2 tablespoons hummus
1 medium cucumber with skin, sliced
8 ounces water or iced green tea with lemon

DINNER
1 serving **Best Bison Burger** (page 115)
1 tablespoon low-sugar barbecue sauce
1 large tomato slice
2 pieces romaine lettuce
1 red onion slice
1 whole-grain thin sandwich bun
1/2 cup fresh raspberries or 1 (2-inch) wedge cantaloupe
4 ounces red wine
Water or tea

DAY 3
1,240 calories

BREAKFAST
1 ounce lox or smoked salmon
1 large egg, soft- or hard-boiled
1 slice whole-grain toast with 1 tablespoon spreadable all-fruit jam
1/2 large pink grapefruit
8 ounces water or green tea with a slice of fresh ginger

MID-MORNING SNACK
1/4 cup fat-free cottage cheese mixed with 1/2 cup salsa
6 baked corn tortilla chips
8 ounces water

LUNCH
1 serving **BBQ Chicken Salad** (page 114)
8 ounces iced green tea or water

MID-AFTERNOON SNACK
1 large apple
1 reduced-fat mozzarella cheese stick
8 ounces spring water

DINNER
1 serving **Roast Pork Tenderloin** (page 134)
2 servings **Warm Cabbage Slaw** (page 137)
1/2 cup steamed brown rice
8 ounces water with fresh lime or green tea

DAY 4
1,140 calories

BREAKFAST
2 servings Baked Ham and Eggs (113)
1/2 toasted whole-grain English muffin
2 tablespoons all fruit spread
8 ounces green tea, water or fat-free milk

MID-MORNING SNACK
1/2 turkey sandwich: 1 slice whole-grain bread, 1 ounce lean sliced turkey,
1 teaspoon mustard
1 large tomato slice, 1/4 avocado
8 ounces iced green tea or water

LUNCH
1 serving Chicken Vegetable Soup (page 119)
1 sliced tomato with rice wine vinegar and cilantro
1/2 cup fresh raspberries
8 ounces iced white or green tea or water

MID-AFTERNOON SNACK
Smoothie made with 1 cup kefir, 1 teaspoon ground flaxseed,
1/2 cup sliced strawberries and 4 ice cubes
8 ounces water

DINNER
6 large shrimp, grilled
2 cups baby spinach salad with 1/2 cup cherry tomatoes,
dressed with 1 tablespoon extra-virgin olive oil
and fresh lemon juice to taste
1 medium peach or pear
4 ounces white wine
8 ounces water or green tea

DAY 5
1,230 calories

BREAKFAST
Breakfast Sandwich: 1 toasted whole-grain thin sandwich bun
    1 egg any style - scrambled, poached, fried
    1 slice Canadian bacon
    1 slice reduced-fat cheddar cheese
    1 cup fat-free milk
    1/2 cup diced melon or watermelon
    Coffee or tea

MID-MORNING SNACK
1 serving **Chocolate Coconut Silk** (page 121)
8 ounces mint tea or water

LUNCH
1 serving **Curried Chicken Salad** (page 124) with 1 cup baby spinach
with 1/4 avocado and 1/4 cup cherry tomatoes
1 small banana
8 ounces iced green tea with lemon or water

MID-AFTERNOON SNACK
1 (2-inch) cantaloupe wedge wrapped with 1-ounce sliced turkey breast
8 ounces water or green tea

DINNER
1 serving **Fire-Roasted Chili** (page 127)
1 medium artichoke, steamed
8 ounces water or mint tea

DAY 6
1,157 calories

BREAKFAST
Omelet (1 whole omega-3 egg plus 1 egg white)
with 1/2 ounce smoked salmon, 1 teaspoon fresh dill
and 4 cherry tomatoes
1/2 cup fat-free Greek yogurt with 1 cup fresh blueberries
8 ounces green tea or water

MID-MORNING SNACK
1 medium apple
One serving reduced-fat string (or cheddar) cheese
1 rye Wasa Crispbread or 1 flax cracker
8 ounces water or mint tea

LUNCH
1 serving **Chicken Vegetable Soup** (page 119)
1 plum
8 ounces water or green tea

MID-AFTERNOON SNACK
1/4 cup fat-free plain yogurt with 1 tablespoon chopped pistachios
and 1/4 cup diced kiwi fruit
8 ounces water or iced tea

DINNER
3 ounces grilled salmon with fresh lemon
1 cup roasted Brussels sprouts with 2 teaspoons slivered almonds
1 serving **Cocoa Sorbet** (page 122)
4 ounces white or red wine
8 ounces green tea with mint or water

DAY 7
1,237 calories

BREAKFAST
2 hard-cooked omega-3 eggs
1 serving **Mango Strawberry Smoothie** (page 130)
8 ounces green tea with lemon or water

MID-MORNING SNACK
Mini sandwich: 2 ounces sliced roast turkey or chicken
with 1 tablespoon **Tangy Tahini Sauce** (page 136)
on 1 slice whole-grain bread
8 ounces water or iced tea

LUNCH
4 ounces poached halibut with fresh lime
1 sliced tomato with 1 tablespoon fresh basil
and 1 tablespoon balsamic vinegar
1/2 cup wild rice
1 cup diced honeydew melon
8 ounces fat-free milk, water or iced tea

MID-AFTERNOON SNACK
1 serving **Blueberry Gingerbread with Pistachios** (page 116)
1 cup hot or iced tea
8 ounces water

DINNER
4 ounces grilled chicken with 1 tablespoon low-sugar barbecue sauce
1 cup sautéed spinach with 1/2 cup sliced mushrooms
1/2 cup baked sweet potato
8 ounces green tea, water or fat-free milk

Week 2 Menus

DAY 8
1,230 Calories

BREAKFAST
Breakfast burrito made with 1 medium whole-wheat tortilla,
3 scrambled egg whites, 2 tablespoons fat-free refried black beans
2 tablespoons salsa, 1 tablespoon grated low-fat cheddar cheese
and 1 teaspoon fresh cilantro
1 cup diced watermelon
1 cup fat-free milk
8 ounces water or green tea

MID-MORNING SNACK
1 serving **Icy Spicy Chai** (page 129)
1/2 sandwich on 1/2 thin sandwich bun, 1 ounce sliced ham,
1 teaspoon mustard

LUNCH
Spinach Salad with Smoked Turkey, Pistachios and Currants (page 135)
1 cup fresh raspberries
8 ounces water with lime slices or green tea

MID-AFTERNOON SNACK

1 low-fat cheese stick
1 pear or apple

DINNER
3 ounces roast chicken or turkey
1 serving **Gingered Edamame** with **Fire-Roasted Tomatoes** (page 128)
8 ounces green tea or fat-free milk

DAY 9
1,265 Calories

BREAKFAST
1 poached omega-3 egg
1 serving **Breakfast Bran Muffin** (page 117)
2 pieces lean nitrate-free turkey bacon
1/2 cup fresh blackberries
8 ounces green tea or water

MID-MORNING SNACK
1 serving **Zippy Green Tea** (page 138)
1 cup nonfat plain Greek-style yogurt
with 2 tablespoons **Cherry Vanilla Granola** (page 118)

LUNCH
3 ounces thinly sliced roast pork tenderloin
1 serving **Confetti Quinoa Salad with Pistachios and Currants** (page 123)
1/2 cup sliced tomatoes
1/2 cup raspberries
8 ounces tea or water

MID-AFTERNOON SNACK
3 medium asparagus spears wrapped with 1/2 ounce smoked salmon
8 ounces iced tea or water with lemon

DINNER
4 ounces grilled sea bass
1 medium artichoke, steamed
1 nectarine
8 ounces green tea or fat-free milk

DAY 10
1,250 Calories

BREAKFAST

2 servings **Mediterranean Scrambled Eggs** (page 131)
1/2 medium banana
8 ounces green tea, ice water or fat-free milk

MID-MORNING SNACK
1/2 thin sandwich bun or 1 small whole-wheat pita stuffed
with 1/4 cup hummus, 2 slices tomato and 4 slices cucumber
Water

LUNCH
1 serving Spinach Salad with Smoked Turkey Pistachios
and Currants (page 135)
1 small peach
Iced green tea with lemon

MID-AFTERNOON SNACK
1/2 cup fat-free cottage cheese with 1/2 medium apple, chopped;
2 tablespoons chopped walnuts; and 2 tablespoons chopped celery

DINNER
1 serving **Best Bison Burger** (page 115)
1 serving **Chili Ranch Dressing** (page 120)
1 cup steamed Swiss chard
8 ounces green tea or water with lemon

DAY 11
1,190 Calories

BREAKFAST
1/2 cup (2) scrambled egg whites with 1 teaspoon fresh herbs,
1/4 cup chopped red onion and 1/4 cup sliced mushrooms
2 slices Canadian bacon
1/4 cup fresh sliced strawberries with 3/4 cup fat-free vanilla yogurt
8 ounces green tea with ginger or water with lemon

MID-MORNING SNACK
3 hard-boiled egg whites filled with 1 tablespoon (each) hummus
Water

LUNCH
1 serving **Easy Salmon with Caramelized Onions and Wild Rice**
(pag 126)

MID-AFTERNOON SNACK
1/2 cup fat-free cottage cheese with 1/2 cup tomato salsa

DINNER
1 serving **Curried Chicken Salad (page 124)**
1 thin whole-grain sandwich bun
1 cup watercress or arugula salad
with 1 tablespoon light balsamic vinaigrette
Iced green tea or water with lemon

DAY 12
1,190 Calories

BREAKFAST
2 servings **Baked Ham and Eggs** (page 113)
1 nectarine
8 ounces iced green tea with lemon

MID-MORNING SNACK
1 serving **Mango Strawberry Smoothie** (page 130)

LUNCH
1 serving **Naked Burrito** (page 133)
1 medium orange
8 ounces green tea or ice water with orange slices

MID-AFTERNOON SNACK
2 Wasa Crispbread with 1 ounce lean ham or roast beef
and 1 tablespoon mustard
Iced tea

DINNER
3 ounces grilled turkey breast
1 cup broccoli florets sautéed with 1/3 cup chopped yellow onion
and 1/3 cup sliced mushrooms
1/2 cup brown rice or quinoa
1/2 cup diced watermelon and 1/2 cup fresh blueberries
with 1 teaspoon fresh mint
8 ounces green tea with ginger or water

DAY 13
1,230 Calories

BREAKFAST
2 servings **Mediterranean Scrambled Eggs** (page 131)
1/2 cup diced watermelon
8 ounces green tea with lemon
Coffee

MID-MORNING SNACK
1/2 cup fat-free vanilla yogurt sprinkled
with 2 tablespoons sliced strawberries and 1 tablespoon chopped pecans

LUNCH
2 servings **BBQ Chicken Salad** (page 114)
Iced Tea

MID-AFTERNOON SNACK
1 serving **Chocolate Coconut Silk** (page 121)
Water

DINNER

4 ounces grilled scallops
2 cups wilted baby spinach with 1 teaspoon olive oil,
1 teaspoon balsamic vinegar and 1 teaspoon grated Parmesan cheese
8 ounces green tea with mint and ginger

DAY 14
1,260 Calories

BREAKFAST
1 cup cold whole-grain cereal
1/2 cup fat-free milk
1/2 banana
1/2 cup blueberries
1 hard-boiled egg
Coffee or tea

MID-MORNING SNACK
Smoothie with 1 cup plain fat-free Greek-style yogurt
1/2 teaspoon vanilla
1 tablespoon cocoa powder
3/4 cup sliced strawberries
Stevia (optional)
8 ounces water or green tea

LUNCH
4 ounces grilled tofu or chicken breast
1 serving **Miso Soup with Spinach and Mushrooms** (page 132)
8 ounces iced green tea or water with lemon

MID-AFTERNOON SNACK
1 peach
1/2 ounce almonds (eight)
8 ounces water or mint tea

DINNER
1 serving **Easy Salmon with Caramelized Onions and Wild Rice** (page 126)
1 cup cherry tomatoes sprinkled with 1 teaspoon balsamic vinegar
and 1 teaspoon chopped basil
4 ounces white wine
8 ounces tea with ginger or water with lemon

RECIPES (25)

Baked Ham and Eggs - Makes 6 servings

This is a great way to start your day with a high protein breakfast. It also works well to make these ahead and reheat in the microwave before serving.

Ingredients:
6 ounces very thinly sliced deli ham
1 1/2 cups salsa or chopped grilled veggies
9 large egg whites or 1 cup + 2 tablespoons liquid egg white
or egg substitute (see note)
2 tablespoons chopped fresh cilantro
2 tablespoons grated low-fat cheddar cheese
Cooking oil spray

Note: If using fresh eggs, separate 9 whites into a medium mixing bowl. Add 1/2 teaspoon salt and whisk lightly. Transfer to a liquid measuring cup. Let stand while you prepare the rest of the ingredients.

Preheat the oven to 400 degrees. Lightly coat each cup of a standard-size nonstick muffin pan with cooking oil spray.

Line each muffin cup with 1/2 ounce of the ham. There will probably be a little excess extending from the top of each cup. Spoon 1 tablespoon of the salsa or veggies into each cup. Measure 3 tablespoons of the egg whites or egg substitute (or a whole egg if using) into each muffin cup. (After the first "muffin," you can pour the whites from the liquid measuring cup to the same level as the first muffin cup, rather than measuring 3 tablespoons each time.)

Place the muffin pan in the oven and bake for 10 to 12 minutes, or until the eggs are puffed and the center is set. Carefully remove the baked eggs from the pan and place two muffins on each serving plate.
Garnish with the cilantro and cheese.

• EGG WHITE FACTOID: A large egg white measures about 2 tablespoons. Adding salt will thin the whites slightly and make them easier to measure by the tablespoon.

Nutritional information (per two "muffin" serving):
Calories 80, fat 2 g, sat fat 0 g, cholesterol 15 mg, sodium 370 mg, carbohydrate 2 g, fiber 0 g, sugar 0 g, protein 12 g

BBQ Chicken Salad - Makes 4 servings

I can never get enough barbecue sauce. This crispy, crunchy salad is one of my favorite ways to enjoy it.

Ingredients:
For the chicken:
1 pound boneless skinless chicken breast cut in 1-inch cubes
1/2 cup low-sugar barbecue sauce, divided
1 teaspoon grapeseed or olive oil
For tortilla strips:
2 small corn tortillas
For the salad:
6 cups shredded Romaine lettuce
1 cup cherry or grape tomatoes, halved
1/4 cup red onion, cut in thin julienne
1/4 cup jicama, cut in thin julienne
1/4 cup shredded reduced-fat cheddar or pepper jack cheese
2 tablespoons finely chopped fresh cilantro
1/2 cup **Chili Ranch Dressing** (see page 120)

Marinate the chicken cubes in 1/4 cup of the barbecue sauce, cover and refrigerate at least one hour. In a medium nonstick pan, heat oil over medium high heat. Sauté the chicken in the pan for about 4 minutes or until done, stirring regularly so the sauce doesn't burn.
Place chicken in small bowl and set aside to cool.

Preheat oven to 350 degrees. Stack the tortillas and cut in quarters with a knife or pizza cutter. Cut quarters into thin strips. Place in a single layer on a nonstick baking sheet. Bake for about 10 minutes or until strips are just starting to turn light brown. Strips will crispen as they cool. Set aside

In a large mixing bowl, combine the lettuce, tomato, onion, jicama, cheese and cilantro. Add dressing and toss well. Divide the salad between four plates. Divide the chicken between 4 plates. Drizzle with remaining 1/4 cup barbecue sauce and top with tortilla strips. Pass extra Chili Ranch Dressing, if desired.

Nutritional information:
Calories 260, fat 5 g, sat fat 1 g, cholesterol 15 mg, sodium 290 mg, carbohydrate 21 g, fiber 4 g, sugar 10 g, protein 32 g

Best Bison Burgers - Makes 8 servings

*Adding quinoa to the meat kicks up the protein and keeps them moist.
You can also shape the mixture into a meatloaf and bake it.*

Ingredients:
1 pound ground bison or lean beef
2 cups cooked quinoa (I used red)
1/2 cup quinoa flakes
1/2 cup minced yellow onion
1/2 cup shredded low-fat cheddar or pepper jack cheese
1/4 cup low-sugar barbecue sauce
2 teaspoons minced garlic
2 teaspoons Worcestershire sauce
2 teaspoons chili powder
1 teaspoon dry mustard
1 teaspoon smoked salt

In a large mixing bowl, combine all ingredients well. There will about
two pounds of mixture, or 4 cups. Place mixture into refrigerator for
at least one hour or overnight. Divide mixture into 8 (4-ounce) patties
using about 1/2 cup meat mixture per burger.

Heat a teaspoon of grapeseed oil in a nonstick sauté pan over
medium-high heat. Add the burgers, cover, and cook about 2 minutes.
Watch carefully so the quinoa doesn't burn. Remove the cover, turn the burgers,
reduce the heat to medium-low, cover the pan, and cook until the burgers are
browned and cooked through, about 2 minutes longer.)

Nutritional information:
Calories 200, fat 6 g, sat fat 2 g, cholesterol 35 mg, sodium 400 mg,
carbohydrate 19 g, fiber 2 g, sugar 3 g, protein 16 g

Blueberry Gingerbread with Pistachios - Makes 16 servings
This irresistibly moist cake is flecked with chewy bits of fruit and crunchy toasted nuts.

Ingredients:
2 cups white stone-ground whole-wheat flour
2 tablespoons ground flaxseed
2 teaspoons baking soda
1/4 teaspoon salt
2 teaspoons ground ginger
1 teaspoon ground cinnamon
1/4 teaspoon ground cloves
1/8 teaspoon ground nutmeg
1/3 cup grapeseed or olive oil
2 large eggs
2/3 cup unsulfured molasses
2/3 cup low-fat milk
1 teaspoon pure vanilla extract
1/2 cup chopped dried blueberries
1/4 cup shelled and chopped pistachios

Preheat the oven to 350 degrees. Lightly coat an 8x8-inch baking pan with cooking oil spray. In a bowl, measure the flour, flaxseed, baking soda, salt, ginger, cinnamon, cloves and nutmeg. Set aside. In another bowl, whisk together the oil, eggs, sweetener, milk and vanilla extract.

Make a well in the reserved dry ingredients and pour in the liquid mixture. Stir until just combined. Fold in the fruit and nuts.

Pour the batter into the prepared pan. Bake for 10 minutes. Reduce the oven temperature to 325 degrees and bake for 30 to 35 minutes longer, or until a toothpick used to test doneness comes out clean.

Nutritional information (per serving):
Calories 190, fat 7 g, sat fat 1 g, cholesterol 25 mg, sodium 220 mg, carbohydrate 26 g, fiber 3 g, sugar 12 g, protein 4 g

Breakfast Bran Muffins - Makes 12 muffins

These moist, fiber-loaded bran muffins are a staple in my kitchen. I usually make a double batch and keep some in the freezer. Try using flavored yogurt, or stir in your favorite fresh berries or nuts if you want even more flavor or texture.

Ingredients:
1 3/4 cups wheat bran or oat bran
1 cup white whole-wheat flour
1/4 cup ground flaxseed (see note)
1 teaspoon ground cinnamon
1 teaspoon baking soda
1/4 teaspoon salt
1 cup fat-free plain Greek-style yogurt
3/4 cup low-fat milk
1/2 cup agave nectar or honey
2 tablespoons grapeseed or olive oil
1 large egg
1 teaspoon pure vanilla extract

Note: Grind whole flaxseeds in a clean spice grinder to the consistency of cornmeal.

Position a rack in the center of the oven and preheat the oven to 400 degrees. Lightly coat 12 nonstick muffin cups with cooking oil spray. In a medium bowl, combine the bran, flour, flaxseed, cinnamon, baking soda and salt. Set aside.

In another medium bowl or in a blender, combine the yogurt, milk, sweetener, oil, egg and vanilla extract and stir or blend until smooth. Make a well in the center of the dry ingredients and pour in the liquid mixture. Using a spoon, stir just until combined. Do not over mix.

Spoon about 1/4 cup of batter into each prepared muffin cup. Bake for 14 minutes, or until the tops spring back when pressed gently in the centers. Do not over bake. Cool in the pan on a wire rack for 10 minutes before removing from the cups. Serve warm or cool completely on the rack.

Nutritional information (per muffin):
Calories 170, fat 4 g, sat fat 0 g, cholesterol 15 mg, sodium 180 mg, carbohydrate 30g, fiber 4 g, sugar 12 g, protein 7 g

Cherry Vanilla Granola - About 10 cups or twenty 1/2 cup servings

I love making my own granola because I can make a different variation each time. Be sure to store in the fridge or freezer to keep it fresh and crunchy.

Ingredients:
6 cups old-fashioned rolled oats (not quick cooking)
3/4 cup raw wheat germ, see note
1/2 cup oat or wheat bran
1/4 cup nonfat dry milk powder
2 tablespoons untoasted sesame seeds
3/4 cup honey
1/3 cup grapeseed oil
1 tablespoon pure vanilla extract
1/2 cup dried tart cherries, chopped (or dried blueberries or cranberries)
1/2 cup chopped pistachios or slivered almonds

Note: It is important that the wheat germ is raw and untoasted.
If not, it may burn in slow toasting process

Position rack in middle of oven. Preheat oven to 250 degrees.
Combine first five ingredients in large mixing bowl.

In a small saucepan, combine honey and oil. Stir over moderate heat until mixture is well combined. Do not boil. Remove from heat. Carefully stir in vanilla extract.

Pour honey mixture over dry ingredients and combine well. Spread out on two sheet pans and place in oven for 1 hour, rotating pans and stirring every 20 minutes to ensure even browning.

Add cherries and nuts during last 10 minutes of baking time. Be sure to allow granola to cool completely before storing in an airtight container.

Nutritional information (per 1/2 cup serving):
Calories 210, fat 6 g, sat fat 0 g, cholesterol 0 mg, sodium 5 mg, carbohydrate 33 g, fiber 5 g, sugar 12 g, protein 6 g

Chicken Vegetable Soup - Makes 12 servings
Loaded with fiber, this recipe makes a large batch of soup, which freezes well, too.

Ingredients:
2 tablespoons grapeseed or olive oil
1 cup finely chopped onions
1 cup finely chopped carrots
1/2 cup thinly sliced celery
2 tablespoons minced garlic
1 pound tomatoes, finely chopped,
or 1 can (14.5 ounces) chopped tomatoes
8 cups fat-free chicken or vegetable broth, see note
1 tablespoon chopped fresh oregano (or 1 teaspoon dried)
1 tablespoon chopped fresh basil (or 1 teaspoon dried)
1 tablespoon chopped fresh thyme (or 1 teaspoon dried)
1/2 cup dry quinoa
2 cups finely shredded kale or spinach
2 cups shredded roast chicken
1 1/2 cups cooked white beans, such as cannellini or Great Northern
1/4 cup chopped Italian parsley, for garnish

Note: If using unsalted or homemade stock,
you may wish to add a little salt to taste.

Heat the oil in a 3- to 4-quart soup pot over medium-high heat. Add the onion, carrots and celery and cook for 5 minutes, or until the vegetables are soft, stirring occasionally. Add the garlic and cook for 1 minute longer. Do not brown. Add the tomatoes, broth, oregano, basil and thyme and bring to a boil. Add quinoa and kale; reduce the heat to a simmer. Cook for 20 to 30 minutes longer, or until the quinoa is tender. Stir in the chicken and the beans; simmer for 5 minutes longer. Season with salt if desired. Garnish with the parsley and serve hot.

Nutritional information (per serving):
Calories 140, fat 3 g, sat fat 0 g, cholesterol 20 mg, sodium 350 mg,
carb 15 g, fiber 3 g, sugar 2 g, protein 12 g

Chili Ranch Dressing - Makes 1 cup, or eight 2 tablespoon servings
*Though this dressing was created for the BBQ Chicken Salad (page 114),
it's fantastic on any salad or as a condiment with grilled fish or chicken.*

Ingredients:
3/4 cup plain nonfat Greek-style yogurt
1/4 cup light mayonnaise
1 tablespoon minced onion
1 teaspoon Worcestershire sauce
1 teaspoon Dijon mustard
1 teaspoon lime juice
1 teaspoon garlic
1 teaspoon chipotle purée or your favorite hot sauce
1/2 teaspoon chili powder
1 1/2 teaspoons minced fresh basil or 1/2 teaspoon dried basil
1 1/2 teaspoons fresh minced dill or 1/2 teaspoon dried dill
1/4 teaspoon fresh ground black pepper

Combine the dressing ingredients in jar of blender or bowl of a food processor.
Blend or process until smooth.

Nutritional information (per 2 tablespoon serving):
Calories 40, fat 2 g, Sat Fat 0 g, cholesterol 0 mg, sodium 90 mg,
carbohydrate 3 g, fiber 0 g, sugar 1 g, protein 2 g

Chocolate Coconut Silk - Makes four 1/2 cup servings

I adore pudding. This is so creamy and chocolatey and easy to make - hope you'll love it too.

Ingredients:
1/4 cup unsweetened natural cocoa powder
1/4 cup cornstarch
1/4 teaspoon salt
2 cups unsweetened coconut milk, see note (if you don't like coconut, you can substitute almond milk or regular milk)
1/3 cup to 1/2 cup agave nectar (depending on how sweet you like your desserts)
2 teaspoons pure vanilla extract

Note: I used So Delicious brand boxed unsweetened coconut milk, which has 45 calories per cup.

In a 1-quart saucepan, combine the cocoa, cornstarch and salt. Add just enough of the coconut milk to make a smooth paste. Gradually stir in the agave and the remaining coconut milk. Cook over medium heat, stirring constantly, until the mixture begins to thicken. Remove from heat and stir in the vanilla extract. Pour into 4 serving dishes and cool.

Nutritional information (per serving):
Calories 150, fat 3 g, sat fat 2 g, cholesterol 0 mg, sodium 330 mg, carbohydrate 33 g, fiber 3 g, sugar 22 g, protein 1 g

Cocoa Sorbet - Makes 1 quart, or eight 1/2 cup servings
Chocolate is one of THE most popular cravings. I love to keep a batch of this on hand since I never know when my next craving will strike!

Ingredients:
1 cup natural cocoa powder
1 3/4 cups water; divided
3/4 cup agave nectar
Pinch salt
1 1/2 teaspoons pure vanilla extract

Measure the cocoa into a small saucepan. Slowly whisk in 3/4 cup of the water until the cocoa is dissolved and there are no lumps. Whisk in the agave, salt and remaining 1 cup water. Over medium heat, bring the mixture to a boil, stirring frequently. Remove from the heat and stir in the vanilla extract. Chill in the refrigerator until very cold. Freeze in an ice-cream maker according to the manufacturer's instructions.

Nutritional information (per serving):
Calories 110, fat 1 g, sat fat 0 g, cholesterol 0 mg, sodium 3 mg, carbohydrate 30 g, fiber 4 g, sugar 24 g, protein 2 g

Confetti Quinoa Salad with Pistachios and Currants - 8 servings

This is a gorgeous side dish to serve with grilled chicken or fish. It's also the perfect dish to take to a potluck, since it can be made in advance.

Ingredients:
For quinoa:
1 teaspoon grapeseed oil
1/4 cup minced yellow onion
1 1/2 cups water or vegetable broth or fat-free low-sodium chicken broth
3/4 cup dry quinoa
For dressing:
1 tablespoon balsamic vinegar
1 1/2 teaspoons lemon juice
1 1/2 teaspoons Dijon mustard
2 tablespoons grapeseed oil
For salad:
1/2 cup dried currants
3 tablespoons coarsely chopped pistachios
2 tablespoons chopped fresh basil
2 tablespoons chopped fresh mint
1 tablespoon fresh lemon zest
1/4 teaspoon salt
1/4 teaspoon ground black pepper

Prepare quinoa:
In a quart saucepan, heat oil over medium-high heat. Add onion and sauté for about 3 minutes or until softened. Add the broth and bring to a boil. Add quinoa, stir, reduce heat, and cover. Simmer for about 10 minutes and remove from heat. Let stand, covered, for 5 minutes. Transfer to a mixing bowl to cool.

Prepare dressing:
In a small bowl, whisk together vinegar, lemon juice and mustard. Whisk in oil until emulsified. Set aside.

Assemble:
Add dressing and remaining ingredients to the quinoa and mix well. Serve immediately.

Nutritional information (per serving):
Calories 140, fat 6 g, sat fat 0 g, cholesterol 0 mg, sodium 100 mg, carbohydrate 20 g, fiber 2 g, sugar 7 g, protein 3 g

Curried Chicken Salad - Makes 3 cups of chicken salad or 6 small wraps

This is delicious served in an artichoke, with a lettuce salad, or tucked in a whole grain tortilla. If you already have leftover roast chicken or grilled chicken on hand, you can use that instead.

Ingredients:
For the dressing:
1/3 cup plain nonfat Greek-style yogurt
1/4 cup mayonnaise
2 tablespoons chutney (I used mango chutney)
1 teaspoon lime juice
1 teaspoon curry powder
1/2 teaspoon ground cumin
1/4 teaspoon ground coriander
For the chicken:
1 tablespoon grapeseed or olive oil
3/4 cup diced yellow onion
1 teaspoon chopped garlic
16 ounces boneless skinless chicken breast cut in 1/2-inch thin strips
1/2 teaspoon salt
1/2 cup chopped dried tart cherries or currants or raisins
1/4 cup chopped cashews, toasted
3 tablespoons fresh cilantro, chopped
For sandwich:
6 7-inch whole-grain tortillas (La Tortilla Factory)

In a medium mixing bowl, combine dressing ingredients; set aside.

Heat oil in nonstick sauté pan over medium-high heat. Add onion and sauté for about 4 minutes or until soft and just beginning to brown. Add garlic and cook for one minute longer. Do not brown garlic. Add chicken and cook, stirring frequently, for about 4 minutes or until chicken is just cooked through. Remove from heat and season with salt. Add cooled chicken mixture to the dressing in the mixing bowl. Add cherries, cashews and cilantro. Stir to combine.

To assemble:
Place about 1/2 cup chicken salad on warmed tortilla. Roll up, burrito style. Serve immediately. Equally delicious served without the tortilla

Nutritional information (per 1/2 cup Chicken Salad without the tortilla): Calories 210, fat 6 g, sat fat 1 g, cholesterol 20 mg, sodium 340 mg, carbohydrate 17 g, fiber 1 g, sugar 13 g, protein 20 g

Easy Salmon with Caramelized Onions and Wild Rice
Makes 4 servings
This is a very simple one-dish meal. I usually serve it with a small salad.

Ingredients:
1 tablespoon grapeseed or olive oil
1 large yellow or white onion, chopped
3 carrots, thinly sliced
1 1/2 cups vegetable or fat-free reduced-sodium chicken broth
1 teaspoon dried thyme
1/4 teaspoon ground black pepper
1 pound skinless salmon fillet, cut into four fillets
2 cups warm cooked wild rice

In a large nonstick sauté pan, heat the oil over medium-high heat. Add the onion and cook for 5 to 6 minutes or until onions are soft and just starting to brown. Add the carrots and cook 1 minute longer.

Add the broth, thyme and black pepper. When the broth comes to a boil, reduce the heat and carefully place salmon fillets in pan. Cover and simmer for 8 to 10 minutes or until the salmon is just cooked through. It will depend on the thickness of the salmon.

Divide the rice among 4 shallow soup bowls or plates. Top each with a salmon fillet and spoon broth and vegetables over the fish. Serve hot.

Nutritional information (per serving):
Calories 310, fat 11 g, sat fat 2 g, cholesterol 50 mg, sodium 250 mg, carbohydrate 25 g, fiber 4 g, sugar 4 g, protein 27 g

Fire-Roasted Chili - Makes about 2 quarts, or 8 servings
This recipe is a real crowd-pleaser. I usually make a double batch and freeze half of it for future use.

Ingredients:
2 cups fat-free low-sodium chicken broth, divided
4 ounces (or 3/4 cup) dried tart cherries, chopped
1 tablespoon grapeseed or olive oil
1 cup chopped onion
1 tablespoon fresh chopped garlic
1 pound lean ground bison, lean beef, chicken or turkey
1 roasted red bell pepper, peeled, seeded and cut into 1/4-inch cubes
1 tablespoon + 1 teaspoon chili powder
1 1/2 teaspoons ground cumin
1 teaspoon ground coriander
1 teaspoon dried mustard powder
1/2 teaspoon dried oregano
4 cups diced fire-roasted tomatoes (or two 15.5 ounce cans)
1 1/2 cups cooked black beans (or one 16-ounce can, rinsed and well drained)
1/4 cup cilantro, chopped

Heat one cup of the broth. Place cherries in small mixing bowl. Add hot broth and set aside.

Heat oil in a 4-quart saucepan over medium heat. Add onion and sauté for about 5 minutes or until onion is soft. Add garlic and cook one minute longer. Do not brown garlic. Add meat and cook just until it is no longer pink.

Add roasted bell pepper, chili powder, cumin, coriander, mustard and oregano. Cook mixture over medium-high heat, stirring occasionally for about 2 minutes. Add tomatoes and remaining cup of broth; bring to a boil. Reduce heat and simmer uncovered for about 5 minutes.

Stir in beans, cherries and cilantro. Continue cooking for an additional 2 minutes or until mixture is just heated through. Season with additional salt if desired.

Nutritional information (per serving):
Calories 230, fat 3 g, sat fat 0 g, cholesterol 35 mg, sodium 440 mg, carbohydrate 31 g, fiber 9 g, sugar 12 g, protein 18 g

Gingered Edamame with Fire-Roasted Tomatoes[3] - Makes 6 servings

While this was intended as a side dish, the edamame is such a great protein source that I often enjoy this as an entrée on Meatless Mondays.

Ingredients:
1 tablespoon grapeseed or olive oil
1 cup finely chopped yellow onion
2 tablespoons peeled and finely chopped fresh ginger
1 tablespoon minced garlic
1 can (14 ounces) fire-roasted tomatoes
2 tablespoons low-sodium soy sauce
1/4 cup vegetable or chicken broth
2 cups shelled edamame
3 tablespoons chopped fresh cilantro, for garnish

Heat the oil in a large sauté pan over medium heat. Add the onion and cook, stirring, for 6 minutes, or until soft and translucent. Add the ginger and cook, stirring, 1 minute longer. Add the garlic and cook, stirring, 1 minute more. Do not brown the garlic. Add the tomatoes, soy sauce, broth and edamame to the pan. Bring the mixture to a boil, reduce the heat, and simmer for 3 to 4 minutes, or until the edamame are just cooked.

Divide among 6 serving plates. Serve hot, garnished with the cilantro.

Nutritional information (per serving):
Calories 128, fat 4 g, sat fat 4 g, cholesterol 30 mg, sodium 90 mg, carbohydrate 381 g, fiber 4 g, sugar 6 g, protein 7 g

---

[3]Adapted with permission from "Positively Ageless" by Cheryl Forberg, RD (Rodale)

Icy Spicy Chai - Makes 6 servings

Move over iced tea. This takes a couple extra minutes to measure the spices but it takes refreshment to a whole new level.

Ingredients:
5 cups water
1 cup low-fat milk or unsweetened almond milk
1 teaspoon natural cocoa powder
1 teaspoon ground ginger
1/2 teaspoon ground cardamom
1/4 teaspoon ground cinnamon
1/8 teaspoon ground cloves
4 black tea bags
2 tablespoons chopped mint
2 tablespoons agave nectar (optional)

Combine the water, milk, cocoa, ginger, cardamom, cinnamon and cloves in a 2-quart saucepan over medium heat. Bring to a boil, then reduce the heat. Add the tea bags and mint and simmer for 4 minutes. Remove from the heat and strain.

Sweeten with the agave, if desired. Chai may be enjoyed hot or chilled. Store for 2 to 3 days in the refrigerator.

Nutritional information (per serving):
Calories 20, fat 1 g, sat fat 0 g, cholesterol 0 mg, sodium 22 mg, carbohydrate 3 g, fiber 0 g, sugar 2 g, protein 1 g

Mango Strawberry Smoothie - Makes 2 servings
I always keep frozen fruit in the freezer to make smoothies on the fly. Add a scoop of your favorite protein powder for a great post-workout recovery drink.

Ingredients:
1 cup fresh or frozen mango chunks
3/4 cup fat-free plain Greek-style yogurt
1/2 cup fresh or frozen strawberries

Combine the fruit and yogurt in a blender. Blend until smooth.
Serve immediately.

The extra serving can be frozen and thawed for another time.

Nutritional information (per serving):
Calories 120, fat 0 g, sat fat 0 g, cholesterol 0 mg, sodium 30 mg, carbohydrate 23 g, fiber 3 g, sugar 19 g, protein 8 g

Mediterranean Scrambled Eggs - Makes 4 servings

A few extra ingredients transform ho hum eggs into a dish you can serve for company. Feel free to add your own twists; sun-dried tomatoes, mushrooms, pesto - the variations are endless.

Ingredients:
4 large eggs
6 large egg whites
1/2 teaspoon Italian seasoning
1 teaspoon grapeseed or olive oil
1/2 cup chopped onion
1 clove garlic, chopped
1/2 cup chopped tomato (or 1/2 cup canned fire-roasted tomatoes, drained)
1 cup chopped fresh spinach
Salt and pepper
1 tablespoon Parmesan cheese

In a medium mixing bowl, whisk the eggs and egg whites with the seasoning, just to blend.

Heat the oil in a medium nonstick sauté pan over medium heat. Add the onion and sauté for 3 to 4 minutes or until just starting to brown. Add garlic and heat one minute longer. Do not brown garlic. Add the tomatoes and sauté 2 to 3 minutes or until heated through. Add the spinach and stir just until wilted. Add the eggs, stirring regularly, for about 2 minutes, or until the eggs are nearly set. Season to taste with salt and pepper and garnish with cheese.

Nutritional information (per serving):
Calories 130, fat 6 g, sat fat 2 g, cholesterol 190 mg, sodium 360 mg, carb 5 g, fiber 1 g, sugar 2 g, protein 14 g

Miso Soup with Spinach and Mushrooms - Makes 6 cups

There is something so restorative about a steaming bowl of miso soup on a chilly day. I also like to serve it in a large shallow bowl for dinner, adding a grilled piece of fish and extra greens and mushrooms.

Ingredients:
1 tablespoon grapeseed or olive oil
3/4 cup finely chopped yellow onion
1 tablespoon finely chopped, peeled fresh ginger
4 cups fat-free, low-sodium chicken or vegetable broth
2 tablespoons sweet white miso
4 ounces firm tofu, drained and cut into 1/4-inch dice
1 cup thinly sliced shiitake or brown mushrooms
1 cup fresh spinach leaves, cut in fine chiffonade (see Note)
Garnish: 1 green onion (white and green parts), very thinly sliced

Heat oil in a 2-quart saucepan over medium heat. Add onion and sauté until just starting to brown, about 8 minutes. Add ginger and sauté for 1 minute. Add broth and bring to a boil.

Whisk in miso until dissolved in soup. Add tofu, mushrooms and spinach and simmer for 1 minute.
Serve warm, garnished with green onions.

Nutritional information (per 1 cup serving):
Calories 60, fat 3 g, sat fat 0 g, cholesterol 0 mg, sodium 500 mg, carbohydrate 6 g, fiber 1 g, sugar 2 g, protein 4 g

Note: The chiffonade cut is done by rolling the leaves lengthwise and slicing crosswise into thin slivers.

Naked Burritos - Makes 4 servings

This "salad" has all the flavors and textures of a burrito, without the wrap. Of course, you can always serve it in a warmed whole grain tortilla if you prefer.

Ingredients:
2 cups cooked brown rice (or quinoa)
1/4 cup chopped cilantro
2 tablespoons finely chopped green onion
1 tablespoon lime zest
1 teaspoon chili powder
1/2 teaspoon ground cumin
1/4 teaspoon ground coriander
1 1/2 cups cooked pinto or black beans (or a 15-ounce can rinsed and drained)
2 cups of your favorite salsa, divided
2 cups shredded roast chicken, about 12 ounces
1/2 cup shredded reduced-fat pepper jack or Mexican blend cheese
1/2 cup plain nonfat Greek-style yogurt
1/4 cup chopped cilantro
2 tablespoons chopped green onion

In a medium bowl, stir the rice and seasonings together just until combined. Divide the mixture among 4 shallow bowls or plates. Top each plate with black beans and 1/4 cup of the salsa. Add roast chicken and top with the rest of the salsa. Sprinkle on the cheese, and add a spoonful of yogurt on top. Garnish with cilantro.

Nutritional information (per serving):
Calories 360, fat 3 g, sat fat 1 g, cholesterol 20 mg, sodium, 170 mg, carbohydrate 46 g, fiber 9 g, sugar 2 g, protein 35 g

Roast Pork Tenderloin with Rosemary and Garlic - Makes 4 servings

Pork tenderloin is a very lean cut - it's on par with skinless chicken breast in terms of fat, cholesterol and calories. Once you see how easy this is to prepare (and how delicious), you'll be making it again and again. Do pay attention to the temperature - it will be dry instead of juicy if you overcook it.

Ingredients:
1 pound lean tenderloin, trimmed of any excess fat
1 tablespoon grapeseed or extra-virgin olive oil
1 tablespoon finely chopped fresh rosemary
1/2 teaspoon salt
1/2 teaspoon ground black pepper
1/2 teaspoon garlic powder
1/2 teaspoon onion powder
Fresh rosemary sprigs, for garnish

Preheat oven to 425 degrees. Brush oil over pork. Combine the seasonings in a small bowl and sprinkle evenly over roast.

Place pork on a small nonstick baking dish in preheated oven. Roast for about 20 minutes or until the internal temperature is 160 degrees in the thickest part. Cover with a clean dry towel and let stand 10 minutes before slicing.

Nutritional information (per serving):
Calories 180, fat 8 g, sat fat 2 g, cholesterol 75 mg, sodium 350 mg, carbohydrate 1 g, fiber 0 g, sugar 0 g, protein 24 g

Spinach Salad with Smoked Turkey and Pistachios
Makes 4 appetizer or 2 main course servings
Chewy, crunchy, sweet, tangy, peppery - it's all here.
Everything can be prepped ahead for a quick last minute meal.

Ingredients:
2 cups baby spinach leaves
1 cup arugula
8 ounces shredded or chopped smoked turkey breast
3 tablespoons chopped dried cranberries
2 tablespoons chopped fresh mint
1 large navel orange
2 tablespoons apple cider vinegar
1 tablespoon Dijon mustard
1 teaspoon agave nectar
1 teaspoon horseradish
1/4 teaspoon salt
1/4 teaspoon ground black pepper
1/4 cup grapeseed or olive oil
Salt and ground black pepper
Garnish: 2 tablespoons chopped pistachios, toasted
(or almond slivers or chopped walnuts)

In a large mixing bowl, place the spinach, arugula, turkey, cranberries and mint. Scrub the orange lightly with an abrasive sponge to remove any surface impurities. Rinse thoroughly and dry well. Remove the peel from the orange with a zester or citrus grater. Peel the orange. Cut the orange in half vertically, then slice the halves horizontally into 1/4-inch-thick pieces. Set aside in small bowl to catch any juices.

In a small bowl, whisk together the vinegar, mustard, agave, horseradish, salt, pepper and oil. Add 3 tablespoons of dressing to the salad and toss well.

To assemble: Arrange the reserved orange slices around the outer edge of chilled plates. Mound the salad in the center. Garnish with the nuts. Pass the remaining vinaigrette.

Nutritional information (per serving):
Calories 190, fat 8 g, sat fat 1 g, cholesterol 25 mg, sodium 220 mg, carbohydrate 15 g, fiber 3 g, sugar 9 g, protein 12 g

Tangy Tahini Sauce - Makes 1 cup or sixteen 1 tablespoon servings

I absolutely love tahini, which is a paste made from sesame seeds. This sauce is a great condiment to serve with a chicken sandwich, or on a grilled piece of fish or chicken.

Ingredients:
3/4 cup plain fat-free Greek-style yogurt
1/4 cup tahini (sesame paste)
1/4 cup Dijon mustard
2 tablespoons water
2 tablespoons chopped fresh cilantro
1 teaspoon fresh lime juice
1/2 teaspoon ground cumin

Instructions:
Combine all of the ingredients in the bowl of a food processor or jar of a blender. Process or blend until smooth. Sauce should be the consistency of thick cream.

Nutritional information (per tablespoon):
Calories 27, fat 2 g, sat fat 0 g, cholesterol 0 mg, sodium 55 mg, carbohydrate 2 g, fiber 2 g, sugar 2 g, protein 3 g

Warm Cabbage Slaw - Makes four 1/2 cup servings

This is a perfect side dish for the Roast Pork Tenderloin with Rosemary and Garlic (page 134) but it's also delicious with chicken, fish or even on its own.

Ingredients:
1 tablespoon grapeseed or olive oil
1 medium yellow onion, finely chopped
2 tablespoons minced garlic
2 tablespoons chopped, peeled fresh ginger
3 cups finely shredded green cabbage
1/2 cup grated carrot
1/2 cup chopped fresh cilantro, without stems
1 tablespoon low-sodium soy sauce
Salt to taste

Heat oil in a large sauté pan over medium-high heat. Add onion and sauté until softened, but not colored, 2 minutes. Add garlic and ginger and sauté for 1 minute longer. Add cabbage and stir-fry until cabbage is softened, about 2 minutes.

Remove pan from heat. Add carrot, cilantro and soy sauce. Stir until combined. Season with salt if desired. Serve hot, warm or cold

Nutritional information (per serving):
Calories 70, fat 3 g, sat fat 0 g, cholesterol 0 mg, sodium 60 mg, carbohydrate 9 g, fiber 3 g, sugar 3 g, protein 2 g

Zippy Green Tea - Makes 6 servings or 1-1/2 quarts
Don't forget – four cups of green tea per day kicks up your metabolism by 80 calories[1] – it all adds up!

Ingredients:
6 cups water
1 cup firmly packed fresh mint leaves
3 green tea bags
1/3 cup agave nectar
1/3 cup fresh lime juice
6 lime slices, for garnish

Bring the water to boil in a 3-quart saucepan. Add the mint and tea bags, remove from the heat, and let steep for 5 minutes. Strain. Stir in the agave and lime juice. Serve hot or iced, garnished with the lime slices.

Nutritional information (per serving):
Calories 40, fat 0 g, sat fat 0 g, cholesterol 0 mg, sodium 15 mg, carbohydrate 13 g, fiber 1 g, sugar 1 g, protein 0 g

---

[1]http://ajcn.nutrition.org/content/70/6/1040.full Am J Clin Nutr. 1999 Dec;70(6):1040-5. Efficacy of a green tea extract rich in catechin polyphenols and caffeine in increasing 24-h energy expenditure and fat oxidation in humans. Dulloo AG et al

Appendix 3
Biomarkers

Biomarkers are measurements of conditions or processes that can help us analyze how healthy our bodies are and how well our bodies are moving through the aging process. Biomarkers for skin health, body weight and muscle mass are visible. Other biomarkers of processes such as immune function, blood sugar control, and blood pressure are more subtle. Collectively, these powerful aging biomarkers dictate our longevity and the quality of life we'll enjoy during our later years.

Below is a quick overview of some biomarkers you may want to monitor during your weight-loss journey. Ideally, you will have a baseline measurement taken before you begin. Recheck after six months to one year to follow your progress.

For more information on biomarkers, refer to the book Biomarkers: *The 10 Keys to Prolonging Vitality* by Dr. William Evans and my book, *Positively Ageless*.

Biomarker: Muscle Mass vs. Fat Biomarker

The following are a few of the most commonly used methods for telling you how much of you is fat and how much is lean body mass - muscles, bones and organs.

A tape measure. According to Dr. Rob Huizenga, the sports doc behind NBC's *The Biggest Loser* program (and former team physician to the NFL's Raiders), an ordinary tape measurement of your waist may be the most cost-effective way to follow your fat loss at home. Ask a friend or family member to place a nonmetal tape measure around your waist, exactly parallel to the floor at belly-button level. After you let out a breath, have your helper take two waist circumference readings - do additional readings if these two are more than half an inch different. This measurement coupled with your baseline weight, can be an effective way to track your progress.

Body-fat calipers. This handheld tool is inexpensive, portable and relatively easy to use. However, its reliability is largely a function of the person using it - you want a pro who's familiar with the process to do it. Often, this is a personal trainer, dietitian or gym instructor. For the test, the health professional gently pinches folds of skin at predetermined sites around your body, then measures the width of each fold with the calipers.

Body-fat scale. Many body-fat scales look like typical bathroom scales, but they go beyond measuring weight. These scales estimate body fat, based on the principles of bioelectrical impedance. Your bare feet come into contact with electrodes when you step onto the metal plates on the scale, and a very mild electrical current passes through your lower body. The machine measures the resistance - or impedance - to this electrical signal as it travels through your legs and lower trunk.

Hydrostatic weighing. Based on water displacement, this is a fairly accurate method of determining body fat and lean body mass. The downside is that the equipment is rather expensive and not as widely available as that for other methods. Hydrostatic weighing takes about 30 minutes to complete.

Bod Pod. This machine is a very useful tool to determine lean and fat mass ratios. While hydrostatic weighing uses water displacement, the Bod Pod displaces air to measure your mass and volume, then calculates your whole body density. It is extremely accurate and a very expensive piece of equipment. The machine is calibrated before every use to guarantee an accurate reading. The reading takes less than a minute and is performed twice for accuracy. The Bod Pod is capable of measuring people who weigh up to 500 pounds. Sometimes found in a physician's office, they are increasingly more available in sports clubs and gyms.

CLASSIFICATION	% FAT (FOR WOMEN)
Essential fat (the minimum you need)	10-12
Athletes	14-20
Fitness	21-24
Acceptable	25-31
Obese	32-plus

Biomarker: Strength

Testing your muscular strength is beneficial in finding your baseline to develop an exercise plan that is tailored to your body. It is recommended that this type of testing be performed by a qualified personal trainer. This important information allows for the creation of an optimal starting point for your exercise prescription. With regular follow-up evaluations you will see measurable improvement that can help you stay motivated, especially if the scale stops moving for a few days. (For more information, see Dr. William Evans' book in Resources)

Biomarker: Basal Metabolic Rate (BMR)

To calculate caloric intake and expenditures for losing (or, in some circumstances, gaining) weight, below is the Harris Benedict Equation for calculating your basal metabolic rate and caloric needs.

For most people, it offers a good estimate of daily caloric needs, though it may underestimate your needs if you're very muscular or overestimate them if you're extremely overweight or have a high amount of body fat. These calculations should be used as a guideline.

If you find yourself *consistently* hungry or tired, you may not be taking in enough calories, so increase your calories slightly until you feel better.

1. Multiply your weight in pounds by 4.35. **Write it here:**

2. Multiply your height in inches by 4.7. **Write it here:**

3. Multiply your age in years by 4.7. **Write it here:**

4. Add the numbers you wrote down in Steps 1 and 2, then add another 655. Next, subtract the number you found in Step 3. **Write your final answer here:**

5. The amount of exercise and other movement you do each day plays a role in how many calories you need. Multiply your number from **Step 4** by:

   1.2 - If you get little to no exercise

   1.375 - If you get light exercise 1 to 3 days a week

   1.55 - If you get moderate exercise 3 to 5 days a week

   1.725 - If you exercise vigorously 6 or 7 days a week

   1.9 - If you exercise vigorously more than once a day, or you exercise vigorously daily plus have a physical job

Write your final number down here. This is how many calories you should take in each day:

If you want to lose weight, cut that number by 20%.
If you want to gain weight, increase that number by up to 20%.

Record this information in your **Food and Exercise Journal:**

Today's Date: _____ Your Daily Calorie Goal: _____

Quick Tip: Online or downloadable calculators, like ones from the Mayo Clinic Calorie Counter or WebMD, can help make this complicated process easier. Plus, an added benefit is that these sites are a wealth of reliable information on nutrition, exercise and overall health.

Biomarker: Aerobic Capacity

Like the Strength Biomarker, this is an excellent measurement of your body's biological age. It measures your body's ability to process oxygen in a set amount of time. It is also an excellent indicator of cardiovascular health. Some of us are simply more fit than others, and measurements such as this are helpful in creating the optimal exercise plan for our bodies. A typical aerobic capacity test would measure your heart rate during physical exertion. A sports professional or qualified personal trainer can make this assessment for you before you begin.

Biomarker: Blood-Sugar Tolerance

The Mayo Clinic site <u>mayoclinic.org/diseases-conditions/diabetes/</u> <u>basics/tests-diagnosis/con-20033091</u> lists tests commonly used to diagnose prediabetes and diabetes. Your health care provider will talk with you about what each test means and what levels you should be at. A couple of common tests are listed below:

Fasting glucose test. With this test, you abstain from eating for at least 8 hours. Your health care provider then takes a blood sample (usually first thing in the morning so it should be at its lowest since you haven't eaten in a while).

Oral glucose tolerance test. Prepare for this test by fasting overnight. The next day, you drink an extremely sweet liquid in your health care provider's office and provide a blood sample 2 hours later. This test is less common, but it may be helpful in determining diabetes in people who show symptoms but have normal blood sugar levels when fasting.

At-home glucose monitoring. There are a number of at-home tests available; talk with your health care provider about what kind of testing schedule you should follow and how to properly measure your blood sugar.

Biomarker: Cholesterol/HDL Ratio

According to the American Heart Association, these are the categories of total cholesterol levels (measurements are in milligrams per deciliter of blood, or mg/dL).[28]

CHOLESTEROL LEVEL	CLASSIFICATION
Less than 200 mg/dL	Desirable
200-239 mg/dL	Borderline high risk
240 mg/dL and over	High risk

But those aren't your only important cholesterol numbers. You should also know your LDL and HDL numbers individually. Remember LDL as *LEAST DESIRABLE*. Here's how LDL breaks down.

LDL LEVEL	CLASSIFICATION
Less than 100 mg/dL	Optimal
100-129 mg/dL	Above optimal
130-159 mg/dL	Borderline high
160-189 mg/dL	High
190 mg/dL and above	Very high

The HDL criterion is simple: You want it above 40 mg/dL, since it protects your health by carrying cholesterol out of your system so it can't cause damage.[29] Remember HDL as *HIGHLY DESIRABLE*.

Another way doctors sometimes weigh the risk from your cholesterol is through the cholesterol ratio. Divide your total cholesterol by your HDL. So if your total cholesterol is 180 and your HDL is 35, the ratio is 5.1 to 1. The ideal ratio is 3.5 to 1, so if your total cholesterol is 180, your HDL would be 51. If your cholesterol is too high (or you want to remain at a healthy level), these dietary changes will help guide your cholesterol biomarkers to where they need to be.

Biomarker: Blood Pressure

Blood pressure is one of many factors your doctor can measure that may be increasing your risk of heart disease.

Systolic blood pressure is the pressure that's measured when the heart beats and pumps blood out; diastolic is the pressure between heartbeats. These make up the two numbers you see when your blood pressure is measured, such as "120 over 80."[30, 31]

The National Institutes of Health has issued the following criteria for determining whether your blood pressure is OK or too high.[32]

- Normal: Your systolic is less than 120, and your diastolic is less than 80.

- Prehypertension: Your systolic is between 120 and 139, and your diastolic is between 80 and 89.

- High blood pressure: Your systolic is 140 or higher, and your diastolic is 90 or higher.

These numbers are valid only if you aren't already taking medications to lower your blood pressure and you don't have diabetes. If you do have diabetes, anything over 130/80 means you have high blood pressure.

Biomarker: Bone Density

Your doctor may recommend a test of your bone mineral density as a way to determine the strength of your bones. It can identify osteoporosis or even a milder level of bone loss leading up to it, called osteopenia.[33] Bone-density testing is performed for people at risk of the condition, including:[34]

- Those with a family history of osteoporosis, osteopenia or certain fractures

- People with low body weight

- People who have had a previous fracture, particularly after menopause
- Women who are simply postmenopausal and concerned about osteoporosis

Several different procedures can measure bone density. One technique, called **DEXA (dual energy x-ray absorptiometry)**, is a popular method because it is highly accurate. This test can measure bone density in your forearm, hip, spine and total body. The test takes less than half an hour as the machine scans your body slowly from head to toe.

Another method to identify weakened bones is an ultrasound bone densitometer, a portable machine sometimes found in drugstores and at health fairs. This method is affordable and fairly accurate. However, it's not as thorough as the **DEXA**. It takes a measurement near your heel, where there is a high percentage of the kind of bone most affected by osteoporosis. The results are used to predict future risk of fracture.

In addition to these scans, your doctor may recommend blood and urine tests to help point out the causes of any bone loss that's found. These measure factors including your calcium and vitamin D levels, thyroid function and estrogen, which point to how fast your bones are building up or breaking down.[35]

Appendix 4
Sample Food Journal Page

Sample Food Journal Page		Day/Date
		Calories
Sample Goal		1200
Meal/Time	Food	Calories
	Totals	
	Goal Totals	
	+ / −	

Appendix 5
Shopping Resources

The listings in this appendix tell you where you can find many of the ingredients called for in this book. Happily, many of these items are more widely available and easier to find than ever before. If you can't find something at the grocery store, always check out your local health food stores, ethnic food shops, and farmers markets, as well. Although this book was written using the most recent research available, new food sources are being established constantly. For updates, go to cherylforberg.com.

Dairy

Cabot Creamery
Products include regular and reduced fat cheeses, plain and flavored Greek yogurt, cottage cheese, and whey protein. Go to cabotcheese.coop to learn about their products and practices. Cabot Creamery 193 Home Farm Way Waitsfield, VT 05673   (888) 792-2268

Redwood Hill Farm & Creamery
Products include natural goat milk yogurt, kefir and cheese, as well as a line of organic dairy products. Go to GreenValleyLactoseFree.com to learn more about the company's products and practices. 2064 Gravenstein Highway North, Building 1, Suite 130, Sebastopol, CA 95472. 707-823-8250 or redwoodhill.com

Organic Valley
A source for cow's milk produced by family farmers without antibiotics, synthetic hormones or pesticides, all Organic Valley dairy farms are pasture-based, meaning a major portion of the cows' diet comes from certified organic pasture. Go to the website for a listing of retail stores where products are sold. Organic Valley Family of Farms CROPP Cooperative, One Organic Way, La Farge, WI 54639. 888-444-6455 or organicvalley.coop/products/milk

Sargento
A Wisconsin-based maker of authentic block, sliced, shredded cheese and cheese sticks. Their wide varieties of cheese are available in full, reduced and/or low fat forms. For more information, on their products and practices, please visit www.sargento.com

Fruits and Vegetables

United States Department of Agriculture's Agricultural Marketing Service
The USDA's searchable directory of farmers markets now includes more than 6,000 listings. It also includes listings for groceries that supply organic produce and information about Community Supported Agriculture programs, explained in the next item on this list. search.ams.usda.gov/farmersmarkets

Community Supported Agriculture (CSA)
These programs put you directly in touch with local farmers by providing a regular (weekly, biweekly, or monthly) allotment of fresh, seasonal produce from their fields, which you can either pick up yourself or, with some CSAs, opt to have delivered to your home. CSAs are growing in popularity and can be an economical way to buy produce. If a weekly box contains too much food for you to use, consider splitting the loot with a friend or two. For more information, go to these sites:

www.nal.usda.gov/afsic/pubs/csa/csa.shtml This USDA site includes helpful links to CSA listings and local farm finders.

localharvest.org/csa Helpful tips for would-be CSA members, including how to select a program and a searchable database of local CSAs.

Farmers Market Coalition
This site for market managers and workers includes state-by-state resource listings: farmersmarketcoalition.org

Local Harvest
This site identifies locally grown produce anywhere in the country. Just click on the map to locate farmers markets, grocery co-ops, CSA, wholesale suppliers and more: localharvest.org

Melissa's/World Variety Produce, Inc.
In addition to selling fresh organic and exotic fruits and vegetables, Melissa's supplies dried mushrooms and other dried produce, herbs, organic agave nectar, whole grains, organic food products and nuts. Go to the website for direct online ordering. P.O. Box 514599, Los Angeles, CA 90051. 800-588-0151 or melissas.com

General and Specialty Foods

Dagoba Organic Chocolate
Products include a collection of 12 chocolate bars infused with pure and exotic flavors, individually wrapped tasting squares, organic drinking chocolate, and baking products. Go to the website for a listing of retail stores where products are sold as well as direct online ordering.
DagobaChocolate.com

Dean & DeLuca
New York-based specialty purveyor offers chocolate, chipotle chilies, crystallized ginger, smoked salt, spices, oils, tahini, teas and coffees. The website offers direct online ordering as well as a listing of retail outlets. 560 Broadway, New York, NY 10012. 800-221-7714 or deandeluca.com

Eden Foods
Products include Japanese sea vegetables, teas, miso, shoyu, rice vinegar, mirin and nori. Also available are fresh-milled whole-grain flours, sesame salts, unrefined vegetable oils, vinegars, tamari, soy sauces, roasted almonds and seeds, packaged snacks, whole grains, quinoa, kosher quinoa, sea salt and popcorn. edenfoods.com

Kalustyan's
This fine-foods merchant offers quinoa, spices, teas, tahini, legumes, sauces, salts and more. Go to the website for direct online ordering. 123 Lexington Avenue, New York, NY 10016. 212-685-3451 or kalustyans.com

Penzey's Spices
Here you can find a comprehensive catalog of herbs, spices and seasonings, including sumac, crystallized ginger and a variety of curry powders, along with unsweetened natural cocoa powders. The website offers direct online ordering as well as a listing of retail outlets. 12001 W. Capitol Drive, Wauwatosa, WI 53222. 800-741-7787 or penzeys.com

Salute Santé
Products include grapeseed oil and infused oils. The website offers direct online ordering. grapeseedoil.com

Scharffen Berger

Products include 41 percent extra-rich milk to 82 percent extra-dark chocolate bars, individually wrapped tasting squares, chocolate baking bars and chunks, and unsweetened and sweetened natural cocoa powder. Go to the website for a listing of retail stores where products are sold as well as direct online ordering. ScharffenBerger.com

The Spice House

This Chicago-area merchant offers a comprehensive catalog of herbs and spices, including sumac, crystallized ginger, and a variety of curry powders. The website offers direct online ordering as well as a listing of retail outlets. 1941 Central Street, Evanston, IL 60201. 847-328-3711 or thespicehouse.com

Grains, Nuts and Legumes

Annie Chun's

Products include quick multigrain rice, black rice and Asian sauces (some contain gluten). The website includes a listing of retail stores where products are sold as well as direct online ordering. P.O. Box 911170, Los Angeles, CA 90091. anniechun.com

Bob's Red Mill Natural Foods

Products include whole-grain flours, quinoa flour, gluten-free oats and gluten-free oat flour, gluten-free baking mixes, seeds, beans and bulk grains. The website includes a listing of retail stores where products are sold as well as direct online ordering. 5000 SE International Way, Milwaukie, OR 97222. 800-349-2173 or bobsredmill.com

King Arthur Flour

Products include whole-grain, nut and gluten-free flours, gluten-free products, ingredients, mixes, tools, and recipes. The website includes a listing of retail stores where products are sold as well as direct online ordering. 135 U.S. Route 5 South, Norwich, VT 05055 800-827-6836 kingarthurflour.com

Living Tree Community Foods

Products include nuts, nut butters (including organic almond butter), oils, agave nectar, honey, flaxseed, almond oil and chocolates. The website offers direct online ordering. P.O. Box 10082, Berkeley, CA 94709. 800-260-5534 or livingtreecommunity.com

The Nut Factory
Products include nuts in their shells: pistachios walnuts, almonds, filberts and Brazil nuts. The website offers direct online ordering. P.O. Box 815, Greenacres, WA 99016. 888-239-5288 or thenutfactory.com

Nuts Online
Products include nuts in their shells (walnuts, almonds, filberts, Brazil nuts, pecans, pistachios and peanuts) along with flaxseed and other seeds, dried fruits, teas and nut butters. The website offers direct online ordering. 125 Moen Street, Cranford, NJ 07016. 800-558-6887 or nutsonline.com

Rancho Gordo
Supplier of heirloom beans and other legumes, chilies, spices, herbs and quinoa. The website includes a listing of retail stores where products are sold as well as direct online ordering. 1924 Yajome Street Napa, CA 94559. 707-259-1935 or ranchogordo.com

Pacific Natural Foods
Products include organic almond, rice and hemp milks; soy milk; and teas, soups and stock. The website includes a listing of retail stores where products are sold as well as direct online ordering. 19480 SW 97th Avenue, Tualatin, OR 97062. 503-924-4570 or pacificfoods.com

Meat, Poultry, and Fish

Alaskan Harvest
Products include sustainably harvested wild ivory king salmon; king, silver and sockeye salmon; and Alaskan black cod available year round. The website offers direct online ordering. 8040 SE Stark Street, Portland, OR 97215. 800-824-6389 or alaskanharvest.com

Organic Prairie
Products include organic beef, pork, poultry and sausages. The website offers direct online ordering. CROPP Cooperative One Organic Way, La Farge, WI 54639. 888-444-6455 or organicprairie.coop

Vital Choice Seafood
Products include sustainably harvested wild salmon, sablefish, scallops, tuna and more. The website offers direct online ordering. P.O. Box 4121, Bellingham, WA 98227 800-608-4825 or vitalchoice.com

Wild Planet
Products include sustainable canned shrimp, tuna, salmon and sardines. The website offers direct online ordering. 1585 Heartwood Drive, Suite F, McKinleyville, CA 95519. 800-998-9946 or wildplanetfoods.com

Sweeteners

Sohgave!
This site offers USDA-certified organic agave nectar and flavored agave nectars. sohgave.com

Wholesome Sweeteners
Products include organic and fair-trade agave nectar, honey, molasses and sugars. The website includes a listing of retail stores where products are sold as well as links to outlets for direct online ordering. 8016 Highway 90-A, Sugar Land, TX 77478. 800-680-1896 or wholesomesweeteners.com

Cooking Equipment and Supplies

Le Creuset
A French cookware manufacturer known for its colorful cookware, bakeware, dinnerware and utensils. Lecreuset.com

The Big Green Egg
Big Green Egg produces high quality ceramic cooking systems for grilling and smoking. Accessories include baking stones, pizza stones and other grilling equipment. To find a dealer, go to biggreenegg.com/locator

WEBstaurant Store
This store is an online source for Squeeze Bottles, baking supplies, measuring cups, cookware and more. webstaurantstore.com

Zeroll Products

Zeroll has a great line of ice cream scoops and spades. Their universal dishers are what I refer to in my recipes as scoops. My favorite sizes are 0.5 ounce (1 tablespoon), 1 ounce (2 tablespoons), and 2.1 ounce (1/4 cup). I also like its Ussentials collection, a line of more than 50 kitchen tools available in a variety of vibrant colors. 3405 Industrial 31st Street, Fort Pierce, FL 34946. 800-USA-5000 zeroll.com

Gluten-Free Resources

Supermarket Savvy

A newsletter and resources to assist you in shopping for gluten-free foods – tip sheets, brand-name shopping lists, comparison charts, presentation kits, supermarket tour kits and kitchen check-ups. The website offers a free virtual supermarket, shopping tips and a complete list of products and services with online ordering. Linda McDonald, MS, RD. Phone: 888-577-2889 or supermarketsavvy.com

The following supermarkets offer gluten-free shopping lists:

√ Ingles Markets: http://www.ingles-markets.com/inside/gluten-free

√ Kroger: kroger.com (search for "Gluten-Free Product List")

√ Meijer: meijermealbox.publishpath.com (Click on the "Healthy Living" tab)

√ Wegman's: wegmans.com (search for "gluten-free products)

√ Whole Foods: wholefoodsmarket.com (click on the "Healthy Eating" tab, then "Special Diets." The site also offers find instructions on gluten-free baking.)

Resources

Evans, William, Irwin H. Rosenberg, and Jacqueline Thompson. Biomarkers: The 10 Keys to Prolonging Vitality. New York: Simon & Schuster, 1992. Print.

Forberg, Cheryl. Cooking with Quinoa for Dummies. Mississauga, ON: J. Wiley & Sons Canada, 2013. Print

Forberg, Cheryl. Positively Ageless: A 28-day Plan for a Younger, Slimmer, Sexier You. Emmaus, PA: Rodale, 2008. Print.

Kramer, Jennie J., and Marjorie Nolan Cohn. Overcoming Binge Eating for Dummies. N.p.: n.p., n.d. Print.

Web Resources

For More on Eating Disorders:
anad.org/get-information/about-eating-disorders/eating-disorders-statistics/

For More Information on Food Addiction and Treatment:
foodaddictioninstitute.org

To Find a Personal Trainer Near You:
IDEA Health & Fitness Association (ideafit.com/find-personal-trainer)

To Find a Nutritionist or Dietitian Near You:
http://www.eatright.org/programs/rdnfinder/

Calorie Counter Apps:
myfitnesspal.com

Online Body Mass Index (BMI) Calculators:
mayoclinic.org/bmi-calculator/itt-20084938

Online Basal Metabolic Rate (BMR) Calculators:
traineo.com/basal-metabolic-rate-calculator

References

1. gallup.com/poll/150986/Lose-Weight-Americans-Rely-Dieting-Exercise.aspx
2. huffingtonpost.co.uk/2012/03/20/average-woman-61-diets-age-45_n_1366665.html
3. mayoclinic.org/healthy-living/weight-loss/in-depth/metabolism/art-20046508?pg=1
4. Lyrics from "You Can't Rollerskate in a Buffalo Herd" by Roger Miller (1965)
5. researchgate.net/publication/51124395_Focusing_on_food_during_lunch_enhances_lunch_memory_and_decreases_later_snack_intake
6. Kong, A. Journal of the Academy of Nutrition and Dietetics, July 13, 2012
7. helpguide.org/life/emotional_eating_stress_cravings.htm
8. webmd.com/diet/features/emotional-eating-feeding-your-feelings?page=2
9. Whole Living, June 2012, citing a study done by the University of Waterloo Dec 2011
10. foodaddictioninstitute.org/scientific-research/physical-craving-and-food-addiction-a-scientific-review/
11. Overcoming Binge Eating for Dummies by Jennie Kramer MSW LCW and Marjorie Nolan Cohn MS RD ACSM-HFS   (Wiley 2013)
12. Mortality in Anorexia Nervosa. American Journal of Psychiatry, 1995; 152 (7): 1073-4.
13. Characteristics and Treatment of Patients with Chronic Eating Disorders, by Dr. Greta Noordenbox, International Journal of Eating Disorders, Volume 10: 15-29, 2002.
14. The Renfrew Center Foundation for Eating Disorders, "Eating Disorders 101 Guide: A Summary of Issues, Statistics and Resources," 2003.
15. American Journal of Psychiatry, Vol. 152 (7), July 1995, p. 1073-1074, Sullivan, Patrick F.
16. The National Institute of Mental Health: "Eating Disorders: Facts About Eating Disorders and the Search for Solutions." Pub No. 01-4901. Accessed Feb. 2002.
17. National Association of Anorexia Nervosa and Associated Disorders 10-year study, 2000
18. The Renfrew Center Foundation for Eating Disorders, Eating Disorders 101 Guide: A Summary of Issues, Statistics and Resources, 2003.

19. Prevention of Eating Problems with Elementary Children, Michael Levine, USA Today, July 1998.

20. Ibid.

21. ajcn.nutrition.org/content/70/6/1040.full Am J Clin Nutr. 1999 Dec;70(6):1040-5. Efficacy of a green tea extract rich in catechin polyphenols and caffeine in increasing 24 h energy expenditure and fat oxidation in humans. Dulloo AG et al

22. Forberg, Cheryl. Cooking with Quinoa for Dummies. Mississauga, ON: J. Wiley & Sons Canada, 2013. Print

23. National Vital Statistics Report, Volume 1, Number 6 dated October 10, 2012. U.S. Department of Health and Human Services, Centers for Disease Control and Prevention.

24. The Fidget Factor Easy Ways to Burn up Calories, Frank I. Katch, Victor L. Katch (Andrews McMell Publishing 2000)

25. Mayo clinic online, staff article mayoclinic.com/health/exercise-intensity/SM00113

26. ewg.org/foodnews/list.php#

27. http://ajcn.nutrition.org/content/70/6/1040.full Am J Clin Nutr. 1999 Dec;70(6):1040-5. Efficacy of a green tea extract rich in catechin polyphenols and caffeine in increasing 24-h energy expenditure and fat oxidation in humans. Dulloo AG et al

28. What Are Healthy Levels of Cholesterol? www.americanheart.org/presenter.jhtml?identifier=183

29. Ibid.

30. High Blood Pressure, www.mayoclinic.com/health/high-blood-pressure/DS00100/DSECTION=2

31. What Is High Blood Pressure? www.nhlbi.nih.gov/health/dci/Diseases/Hbp/HBP_WhatIs.html, americanheart.org/presenter.jhtml?identifier=4756

32. High Blood Pressure, www.mayoclinic.com/health/high-blood-pressure/DS00100/DSECTION=2

33. National Osteoporosis Foundation, nof.org.

34. National Institute of Arthritis and Musculoskeletal and Skin Diseases http://www.niams.nih.gov/health_info/bone/Bone_Health/bone_mass_measure.asp

35. Ibid.

ACKNOWLEDGMENTS

This book is the result of countless collaborators and friends who contributed valuable insights, shared their expertise, and simply lent their support and enthusiasm.

Of course, this book would not have been possible without the tireless and thorough work of my team at Flavor First LLC, especially Sandee McCready, who shaped and co-wrote the manuscript while providing valuable feedback along the way. You helped bring my words to life while never losing sight of the big picture - thank you, Sandee!

As well, technical reviewer (and dear friend) Susan Bowerman, MS, RD, made certain that everything in this book was precise and accurate. Thanks to Cheryl Kurowski, MS, RD, my fabulous research dietitian, and to Moira Allison and Anita Anim, RDs to-be and social media interns extraordinaire – thank you!! And to my sister, Paula Beritzhoff for your wit, advice, support, and for always believing in me.

I am indebted to my agent and good friend, Jim Molesky, for his support and belief in this project and all of my work – thank you, Jim!

Many thanks to the incredible team at Shine and *The Biggest Loser* family including: Vivi Zigler, Monica Austin, Kelia Tardiff, Whitnee Null, Edwin Karapetian – to our incredible trainers, Dolvett Quince, Jen Widerstrom, Jessie Pavelka, Bob Harper and Jillian Michaels! To our amazing production team including Joel Relampagos, Dave Broome, Alex Katz, Annie Imhoff, Will Erb, Kat Elmore, Kristen Mearns, Kelsey Schneider and so many more! And to my colleagues on the Medical Expert team at *The Biggest Loser*, Dr. Rob Huizenga, Dr. Marc Boff and Dr. Sean Hogan – thank you all so much for your continued support of my work on *The Biggest Loser*!

The supportive community of registered dietitians continues to inform and inspire me. My friends and colleagues at the American Dietetic Association, especially the Food & Culinary Professionals group, have provided invaluable guidance to me throughout my career.

My sincere appreciation goes out to the many companies and individuals who provided technical and product support for the recipes that went into this book. Chief among these are Fisher & Paykel Appliances, who provided the gorgeous media kitchen in which my recipes were developed; KitchenAid for my countertop appliances; Le Creuset for the beautiful and sturdy dishes and cookware we used; and Zwilling J.A. Henckels for cutlery and non-stick pans. A special thanks also goes out to Debra Cohen and Melissa's Specialty Produce, who supplied much of the produce for my recipe development, and to the American Pistachio Growers for their support of my work and the generous supply of pistachios!

My personal trainer, Ines Donnelly of NapaFit, is my inspiration for this book which she has been requesting for years.

To all of my friends at Omni Hotels & Resorts, especially David Morgan, Anne Tramer, Molly Phillips, and Brandon Smulyan – thank you for your continued support and friendship. I love working with you!

To my many friends who offered their constant support, kindness, and humor, and, perhaps most importantly, their palettes for impromptu tastings. Thanks to Claudia Sansone Hampton and Melissa Roberson for their friendship and guidance. and to Dowl, Amelia, and Taylor Hollabaugh, for being my recipe tasters. To Karen and Steve Price, Paula and John Beritzhoff, Patricia Treible and especially Paul Skittone – thank you for keeping me sane throughout the process and patiently enduring my crazy schedule.

Most of all, to Mom – thanks for your endless love, encouragement and support – and for always being there.

INDEX

Daily Calorie Budget	
Calories per meal	
Calories per snack	
Protein calories per day	
Protein grams per meal	
Protein grams per snack	

NOTES